THE ESSENTIAL OILS DIET

*Lose Weight and
Transform Your Health
with the Power of Essential
Oils and Bioactive Foods*

ERIC ZIELINSKI, DC,
AND **SABRINA ANN ZIELINSKI**

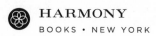 **HARMONY**
BOOKS · NEW YORK

Copyright © 2019 by DrEricZ.com LLC

All rights reserved.
Published in the United States by Harmony Books,
an imprint of the Crown Publishing Group, a division of
Penguin Random House LLC, New York.
crownpublishing.com

Harmony Books is a registered trademark, and the
Circle colophon is a trademark of Penguin Random House LLC.

Library of Congress Cataloging-in-Publication Data is available upon request.

ISBN 978-1-9848-2401-1
Ebook ISBN 978-1-9848-2402-8

Printed in the United States of America

Book design by Elizabeth Rendfleisch
Illustration by iStock.com/filipfoto
Jacket design by Jessie Sayward Bright
Jacket photographs: (lemon) Viktor1/Shutterstock; (mint) GCapture/Shutterstock; (grapefruit) Flaffy/Shutterstock

10 9 8 7 6 5 4 3 2 1

First Edition

To Esther, Isaiah, Elijah, and Isabella: You are our gifts from the Lord, and we love and appreciate you more than you'll ever know. You have helped us experience and understand the love of God in a way that no one else could ever explain, and being your parents has helped complete us.

We trust that you will see this book as our family's gift to the world, and that you will consider the time that we sacrificed away from each other as we prepared the manuscript worth it in the end. This is why we do what we do and the reason why we live the way that we do. You are our inspiration and the hope for a healthier generation that will experience the abundant life!

Love,
Daddy and Mommy

CONTENTS

MEET THE ELEPHANTS IN THE ROOM

*"The greatest revolution of our generation is the discovery
that human beings, by changing the inner attitudes of their
minds, can change the outer aspects of their lives."*
—WILLIAM JAMES

Fair warning: There are two reasons this is unlike any diet book you
have read before.

- Reason #1: To our knowledge, this is the first book that
  describes using bioactive compounds such as essential oils to
  control your weight and help prevent disease. Most likely you
  have not heard of "bioactive compounds" before, although I'm
  sure that you're familiar with such terms as *antioxidants* and
  even *polyphenols*. Both are bioactives, which should be the real
  focus of your diet program. Don't worry, we'll cover this in
  depth later on.
- Reason #2: Food is neither at the core of the problem nor is it
  the solution. The real issue is something totally different: Why
  do people fall prey to behavior that they know in their heart
  of hearts is bad for them? And more importantly, how do
  you escape that trap and transform your life? That is the real
  subject of this book.

Every year dozens of new diet books debut, several of which wind
up on bestseller lists. Turn on the television or pick up a magazine and

you will likely see advertisements for weight-loss programs, complete with meals delivered to your doorstep. Americans are obsessed with dieting, but if you look around, it is clear that, as individuals, we are spectacularly unsuccessful at achieving the goal of a healthy weight. Even worse, we are exporting the American way of eating to the rest of the world, with predictable consequences.

Our addiction to food is matched by our addiction to diets. We might as well be seeking the fountain of youth instead of remaining youthful longer by changing our ways. The reality is that most diets don't work, but the fantasy remains that if we can only find the right book with the right diet, we will be transformed and live happily ever after. But we have it backward: commit to changing your life, and you can start down the path that leads to the transformation of your health and your body.

Now I know you are thinking: "Wait a minute: This book contains the word *diet* in the title, so why are you talking out of both sides of your mouth?"

Unfortunately, the word *diet* has been co-opted by the weight-loss industry. Originally, *diet* simply referred to a way of eating, but now most people associate the word with weight loss. In this book, *diet* refers to its original meaning, specifically to a way of eating composed of bioactive-rich foods full of essential nutrients and the parallel elimination of processed foods. As you'll learn, weight loss is a side effect of eating well and adopting other healthful habits.

Abundant Life: Your God-Given Right

"The thief comes only to steal and kill and destroy. I came that they may have life and have it abundantly."
—JOHN 10:10

In my last book, I asked if readers considered themselves to be healthy. I quoted the World Health Organization's (WHO) definition of *health* as "a state of complete physical, mental and social well-being and not merely the absence of disease or infirmity," and I challenged them to think beyond what they may have considered *health* to be: a truly vibrant, abundant life that is infinitely more than just the absence of sickness and disease.

In this book, I'd like to take that discussion one step further and ask you a different question: Do you enjoy an *abundant life*? In other words, are you enjoying biblical health?

Biblical health is not a list of "thou shalt nots." Rather it's an overarching concept that it is your God-given right to have and enjoy the abundant life that Christ refers to in John 10:10. This means that you enjoy balance and manifest health in all areas of your life: spiritual, physical, mental, emotional, financial, occupational, and social. Stay tuned, we'll discuss most of these seven areas in greater detail and will give you tips on how to master them in chapter 9.

Your Health Is the Cornerstone

Most books and teachings designed to help you achieve the abundant life do so by focusing on prayer, meditation, acts of service, and other spiritual practices. Although these are all good and necessary methods, they miss the fundamental fact that your health is truly the cornerstone of your life. This book focuses on the practical truth that a balanced and abundant life is impossible if your physical body becomes a burden to your soul.

Again, let me ask: Do you enjoy an *abundant life*?

I encourage you to start a journal as you embark on this journey with us—think of it as your Transformation Journal—and write your answer to that question inside the front cover. As you read this book, go back to this question again and answer honestly. Remember, at its core, your health journey is about balance. The foods you eat, the drinks you consume, the supplements you take, the medicines you use, the thoughts you think, the emotions you carry around, the feelings you have about your job, your financial practices, and the stressors that you allow in your life—all of these contribute to or diminish your experience of an abundant life. And while you're at it, record your current weight and measurements of your chest, upper arms, waist, hips, and thighs. It will be exciting to watch all those numbers shrink in the coming weeks and months.

Introducing Mama Z

Now a little background. My first book, *The Healing Power of Essential Oils,* set the foundation for how to use essential oils, which are an important component of my approach to the abundant life. This new book is the natural progression, addressing the elusive goal of achieving a healthy weight as integral to good health. This time, I am proud to say, my coauthor is my wife and ministry partner, Sabrina, aka Mama Z.

Together we're going to debunk several myths and set the record straight on some key and timely topics that are relevant to you and your health, one being how those low-carb, high-fat fad diets you hear so much about are not something you should adopt if you're trying to experience an abundant life. Another is that it is important to understand that a slim body is only one aspect of overall health. You can look great but be unhealthy; however, you cannot be truly healthy if you are overweight.

So rather than a traditional "diet" book, you hold in your hands the key to peak health, high performance, and true transformation. Our full intention in writing it is to give you the tools that you need to experience a well-balanced abundant life by first achieving a healthy weight.

In the following chapters, we will address emotional detoxification and body image, help you find the right exercise routines, and provide delicious, quick, and easy recipes so that you can enjoy a long life of abundant health and wellness.

Myths and Misinformation

It is critical that you not blame yourself for either your extra pounds or your health problems. Guilt only compounds self-destructive habits, and any guilt is misplaced. Something has happened that has desensitized your body to the usual cues that signal hunger and satiety. We have all suffered at the hands of such misinformation.

Your parents, your doctors, and your teachers fed you the lie, but they were fed the lie themselves. Most conventionally trained physicians know little about nutrition. The lie is that the American diet is nutritious and the diseases that plague our people have little or nothing to do with the quality of our diet.

Really?

Consider the following facts that as a culture we prefer not to acknowledge. Mama Z and I call them the elephants in the room.

Meet Elephant #1: There's No Oil for That

My first book set the groundwork for how to use essential oils. No sooner was it published to great success than droves of people besieged Sabrina and me, requesting solutions to their health problems. They asked: Which essential oil should I use to deal with diabetes? Which oils can relieve my depression or anxiety? Which oils can eliminate my acid reflux? How about weight loss? And on and on it went with countless other health issues.

They all asked the wrong questions. This assumption that one oil or a combination of oils can itself be a cure is flawed. Don't fall for that trap. The last thing we want to do is to regard essential oils as we do pharmaceutical drugs, as a quick fix rather than lasting change. Oils enhance your body's ability to heal itself and can help improve the experience of reaching your ideal weight. They will not help you achieve lasting weight loss if you're not willing to change your lifestyle, which brings us to our second point.

The simple truth is that no single oil banishes excess pounds.

Meet Elephant #2: Oils Alone Can't Banish Pounds

The simple truth is that essential oils alone cannot solve your weight issue. Only by transforming your lifestyle can you reach your body's natural healthy weight, and we will show you how to use essential oils to make your life a lot easier during the process!

Mama Z and I subscribe to a vitalistic approach to health, which holds that the power that made the body can heal the body. God has given your body the remarkable innate ability to heal itself under the right conditions. No amount of essential oils can heal the body *without other changes.* You can't live on fast food and expect essential oils to enable you to slim down.

Essential oils are known harmonizers, which will *help* your body reach the homeostasis necessary to truly prevent disease and treat sickness. In partnership with changes in diet, mental attitude, exercise, and other lifestyle modifications, essential oils can play a powerful role in helping you achieve and maintain a healthy weight.

Meet Elephant #3: You Cannot Be Healthy if You Are Overweight

The real question you need to ask yourself is this: What lifestyle changes do I need to make to set the stage for optimal health and disease prevention? We live in a world full of environmental toxins. Many of those toxins can be found in the typical American diet of processed foods and fast food. An essential factor in determining your health is your weight. If you are overweight, you cannot be truly healthy. Ditto if you are underweight. And if you are very overweight, your health is even more imperiled. To be truly healthy, you need to achieve your body's natural weight.

Meet Elephant #4: Poor Health and Overweight Are Ballooning

Despite our technological and medical advances, and the billions of dollars we spend as a nation on health care, we are not getting collectively healthier. In fact, the statistics show just the opposite. According to the Centers for Disease Control and Prevention (CDC), 39.8 percent of American adults are obese.[1] Add in merely overweight adults and the number is even more appalling: 70.7 percent, despite the fact that approximately 45 million Americans go on a weight-loss diet each year.[2] Obesity and overweight are linked to heart disease, stroke, type 2 diabetes, and certain types of cancer, which means that all these leading causes of death are in fact highly preventable if people keep their weight down!

The most recent statistics reveal that more than 100 million Americans already have type 2 diabetes or prediabetes, and about half that number is undiagnosed as yet. Of those, 30.3 million have full-blown diabetes, and the remaining 84.1 million have prediabetes. Plus 34 percent of American adults have metabolic syndrome, a cluster of conditions related to diabetes—specifically excess abdominal fat, abnormal cholesterol levels, high blood sugar, and increased blood pressure—that occur together, increasing your risk of diabetes, heart disease, and stroke.[3]

Meet Elephant #5: The Next Generation Is in Deep Trouble

For the first time in history, children are now expected to have shorter lifespans than their parents, thanks in large part to diseases such as type 2 diabetes, elevated blood pressure, heart conditions, and joint deterioration—all conditions linked to obesity.[4] Again, these diseases are largely preventable. There is no question that we are facing a crisis of mammoth proportions, and Mama Z and I are committed to doing our part to put an end to it.

This is why we decided to write this book: to walk people through the easy-to-implement strategies that we have developed over the years to become and stay fit and find a healthy weight, with the support of essential oils. It is our sincere hope that after reading this book you can become a role model for health and transformation and help share our important message with your friends and loved ones.

Let's begin. . . .

HOW DID WE GET INTO THIS MESS?

"You can't have a physical transformation until
you have a spiritual transformation."
—CORY BOOKER

Consider these facts:

- Our food is laced with a barrage of additives, preservatives, and other chemicals, many of which have never been tested on humans. The jury is still out on whether genetically modified organisms (GMOs) are a threat to conventionally grown crops, food animals, and humans.
- Even chemicals that have been tested have not been tested over a normal lifetime. Both the Food & Drug Administration (FDA) and the US Department of Agriculture (USDA) are heavily funded by the pharmaceutical, agricultural, and chemical industries. In effect, we have all become guinea pigs in a gigantic science experiment that spews toxins into our air, water, and food without considering the results.
- According to a 2015 study, four-year medical schools are required to provide a minimum of just twenty-five hours of nutrition education, but only 71 percent of 121 schools that responded to a recent survey actually provide even this meager minimum. The authors of the study concluded, "It cannot be a realistic expectation for physicians to effectively address obesity, diabetes, metabolic syndrome, hospital

malnutrition, and many other conditions as long as they are not taught during medical school and residency training how to recognize and treat the nutritional root causes."[1] No wonder doctors are more likely to prescribe a pill than to explore a patient's eating habits.

- Much of the food fed to the nation's schoolchildren is surplus grain subsidized by the USDA and canned goods, rather than fresh vegetables and fruits, which are too expensive for many school budgets. Kids learn poor eating habits in the very place they should be learning about good nutrition.

The result of this ignorance or misinformation is nothing less than a crisis. As we mentioned in the preface, almost 40 percent of American adults are obese and 71 percent are overweight.[2] Being heavy has become the norm.

Nor is this just a matter of body image and clothing size. Conditions linked to excess weight, including cancer, hormone imbalance, gut disorders, and type 2 diabetes, have also spiraled. Our children are victims of this crisis, too, with obesity rates of 9.4 percent, 17.4 percent, and 20.6 percent for children two to five years old, six to eleven years old, and twelve to nineteen years old, respectively.[3] The older kids are, the likelier they are to be obese. The bad news continues: as more and more cultures adopt the standard American diet (aptly abbreviated as SAD), this crisis is spreading worldwide. We call it a national eating disorder.

The disorder is not confined to the United States. According to the WHO, by 2016 the incidence of obesity had almost tripled since 1975, comprising almost 2 billion overweight adults, of whom more than 650 million were obese. More than 340 million children aged five to nineteen were obese or overweight that same year.[4] The sum result of all this is a national—dare we say international?—eating disorder that is making us sick, fat, and burdened with ballooning medical and pharmaceutical bills.

We firmly believe that this disaster can be rectified one family at a time by following our program.

Tales of Transformation

If it isn't crystal clear from the preface, this book is not about quick fixes such as eating berries, taking probiotics, or using lime oil in your diffuser to improve your health, although we recommend all these natural approaches. Rather, we are talking about total transformation of who you are, how you live, what you eat, and how you interact with others. Weight loss is a physical manifestation of transformation, and attaining a slim, healthy body will likely inspire you to make other changes in your life. Foods rich in bioactive compounds and essential oils can play important roles in this process, but transformation is manifested in a way of living, of relating to others, even as a spiritual experience.

We hope that our own stories of transformation will inspire you to reshape your life and create your own story.

Dr. Z here. I shared my story of transformation at length in my first book, so I'll give you a brief version now, but my wife and coauthor's transformative experience is particularly applicable to this book, so I want to get to that as quickly as possible.

My childhood was marred by poor health. From birth I was fed formula and cow's milk, which made me excessively plump, so my pediatrician put me on a diet of low-fat milk when I was just a few months old. As a preschooler, I was plagued by tonsillitis, enduring multiple treatments with antibiotics and later a tonsillectomy and adenoidectomy. I also suffered from anxiety and difficulty dealing with stress. By the age of five, I had developed a stammer that required working with a speech therapist. Adolescence brought cystic acne, joint pain, and digestive issues. I was not a happy camper! Then when I went to college, I fell prey to the temptations that sabotage so many college students: partying, drinking, smoking, and doing drugs. Lots of drugs. So much so that I found myself on a five-year binge that is now pretty much a blur to me.

My transformation began when a business associate took me under his wing, allowing me a glimpse into his full and rewarding life. He became an instant father figure for me, and I became one of his "spiritual sons." He wasn't rich, but he made good money, had good relationships, enjoyed good things in life, and was super healthy. I was like, "Man, this is possible." He also introduced me to an abundant life that I had never thought was possible.

As a kid I once thought I was destined for greatness, but something happened along the way, and I started doubting myself. I felt empty, in despair, as though I was looking down a long black tunnel. I realized that even though I knew I was doing bad things to my body, I was doing them anyway. Once you ignore your conscience and common sense, you separate yourself from reality.

However, once I committed my life to Christ at the age of twenty-two, my transformation was immediate. All my bad habits and addictions—snorting cocaine, smoking marijuana and cigarettes, and drinking alcohol—vanished from my heart. Since then, I have not used any of these crutches. Importantly, I also changed the way I was eating. Up until then, I was pretty much on the standard American diet (SAD) and had no idea how to take care of my health.

For me, my transformation was an "I was blind, but now I see" moment. My spiritual awakening rekindled my childhood desire to be a doctor, and I enrolled in chiropractic school. Meanwhile, I continued my career as a public health researcher and writer. Sabrina had been interested in essential oils since childhood, and I appreciated the healing powers of her household and personal concoctions, but it wasn't until I realized how much solid research confirmed their efficacy that I decided to enroll in the long and intensive training necessary to become an aromatherapist. Together, we are now the parents of four wonderful children and share work that we love. God is good!

Now over to my lovely wife.

Mama Z here. In my case, I was trapped in an eating disorder I had suffered with for years. I was allergic to dairy from childhood, and my problems with food grew over the years. I was plagued with digestive issues resulting from undiagnosed food sensitivities and had gotten to the point that there were very few foods that did not disagree with me. At one point I was actually eating only four foods. Dining out was problematic, but because I was in a job that required frequent entertaining, I fell into bulimia. I would eat what was served and then go to the restroom and make myself throw up, because I knew how sick it would make me feel due to my sensitivity to so many foods.

I'd experienced success in other areas, and that gave me a taste of what I could have throughout my whole life. Transformation starts with a choice. And most of the time, that choice comes from reaching a pain point, which may be physical or emotional. When you're no longer willing to deal with the pain, then you're ready to commit to something new. I'll never forget when one of my exercise class students, who was being abused by her husband, said to me, "I knew I was ready to move on when I cared less about the unknown than what I knew I would get in the known. But I had to get to that point before I could change." The same was true for me, although in my case it was food that was giving me pain.

I was raised in faith and I love all the people I met in the church I grew up in, but the very first time a friend invited me to attend a nondenominational church, I felt the presence of God as I never had before. His spirit was alive and on fire. After church, I had lunch with my friend's family and I was like, "Can I go again?" They replied, "We have a service tonight." And I said, "I want to go." And so I went every time the doors opened. I was born again on Easter of 2004, and a few months later I was water baptized, which was an awesome experience.

Part of my healing journey involved a ten-day water fast. During that process I prayed for God's help and I weaned myself off the ten pharmaceuticals doctors had prescribed to deal with my digestive issues, allergies, dysmenorrhea, and ADHD, but my eating disorder was still with me. For years I had asked doctors to test me for food sensitivities without success, so I started doing it myself, by withdrawing a food and then reintroducing it to gauge my response.

As a result of this experimentation, I learned I couldn't eat wheat. Then I realized sugar was a problem when I overdid it and my face puffed up as though I had been sucker punched. No dairy, no sugar, and no wheat rule out most foods. I missed ice cream, so it occurred to me that perhaps I could have a frozen soy-milk version. But I soon realized I was allergic to soy, too. At that time I didn't know what I do now: soy is almost always genetically modified, and it's also one of the crops sprayed most heavily with pesticides. In addition, many people are soy-intolerant as well as lactose-intolerant.

Once I came to grips with my food allergies, I would pray over my hands before I would cook. I would say, "Lord, I know not what I'm doing, but I know you will guide my hands in the kitchen when I have to relearn everything." At first, I thought I would have to start all over again. I didn't realize that I would be able to build on the groundwork of traditional recipes and learn how to modify them.

Eric's transformation was almost instantaneous, but mine was a slower process. I knew there was something more I could do, but I didn't know that it would result from meeting Eric at church and him coming into my life. Our meeting truly transformed my health journey and transformed me in other ways. Early in our relationship, he said, "Let me cook for you." The amazing thing is that all my symptoms went away. I like to tease him that these meals were all brown and green, being mainly composed of grains and greens, but the truth is my bulimia and food disorders resolved. I have since added a rainbow of other colorful foods to our meals!

Despite the fact that I hadn't been eating that much, I was still not able to achieve my ideal weight, but under Eric's guidance and less than a month after cutting out all the foods I was allergic to, I had lost ten pounds. I responded so well that I could eat more than just those four foods and still feel good. Today, as long as I stay away from dairy, sugar, all forms of gluten, soy, table salt, and preservatives, I am okay. And the great thing is that with the tasty substitutes I have found for those problematic foods, I can now enjoy delicious and wonderfully varied meals without endangering my health. I'll be sharing those alternatives in Part 3.

Transformation comes from a deep desire or need, and it is often rooted in pain. In order to make a change, there has to be more motivation than just "I want to lose five pounds to look good in my bathing suit." That's not what's going to get you out of bed at 6 o'clock in the morning to go work out. There's got to be more of a drive.

Much of my drive comes from the five people who depend on me all the time—Eric and our four wonderful children. Of course, I want to be healthy, but I *have* to be healthy for my family. As a couple, Eric and I also need to be healthy and fit so that we can help people in our church and our community be healthy and fit, too. We're not going to give advice to somebody if we're not going to do it ourselves. So everything we talk about and write about in our books and on our website, we do ourselves.

"Take delight in the Lord, and He will give you the desires of your heart" *(Psalm 37:4)*. Now all my desires are for life-giving things, giving myself up to God, living as Jesus did, desiring good things for others, being healthy, feeling joy in the sun's warmth and in the movement of my body. Once you start living your life to delight your Creator and serve others, your heart starts to change. You desire the things that promote healing, spiritual growth, and appreciation of life.

The Path to Transformation

We encourage you to open yourselves up to transformation, and we believe that *The Essential Oils Diet* provides the path. And we suspect that when you experience transformation, you'll find it easy to leave behind your bad food habits. Our hope is that after reading this book, you will not just buy in but also be absolutely convinced that yes, you *can* do this. You *should* do this. And you *will* do this.

A friend of ours, Jason Carver, a well-known trainer in Atlanta and founder of DreamBody Inc., has three questions he asks his clients:

1. Do you want to change? (Always a yes.)
2. Are you willing to change? (Usually the answer is "Yes, but don't make me drink green smoothies" or something similar.)
3. Do you have the confidence and mental drive to implement what it takes to change? (Typically answered with "I hope, or

I think so." They usually tell him that they don't think they can sustain a commitment to a program.)

Jason will only work with people who are totally committed to doing whatever it takes. That is the same level of commitment you will need to follow the Essential Oils Diet.

What Is Your "Why"?

"Do you not know that your bodies are the temples of the Holy Spirit?" *(1 Corinthians 6:19)*. Are *you* willing to do whatever it takes? That's the level of commitment that you need to transform yourself. Is your "why" your family, your spouse, your ministry, your obligation to honor God? Or do you simply want to look and feel better?

We have discovered that people need a significant deep-rooted, life-transforming "why" to enable them to find their ideal weight and enjoy the abundant life. Whether it's our program or any run-of-the-mill low-carb diet book you find on the shelves, you won't have a chance of success if you don't have a determined *why*.

And therein is another of the many reasons why diets don't work. They are usually based on vanity alone. Lose twenty pounds in twenty days, yada yada. That motivation, the desire for a beach body, is not going to last. Transformation is unlikely to happen under such circumstances.

But if you have deeper motives for doing this, whether to become healthy and have the energy to care for your family, serve other people, or serve your God, such motives will propel you through the difficult times. We suggest it be your devotion or moral obligation to a higher power. Trust us, if you stay true to your heart that your body is a temple, you'll find that you have a moral obligation to take care of it. And this will hold you to a level of accountability that nothing or no one else could ever do.

Secondary is our obligation and desire to help our family. And third is to be healthy and look good, which is a good reason, but it should not be the first—and it should not be the only reason. And if you have all three of these reasons, you have just set yourself up for success.

Nor must you be what is usually considered a religious person to do this for a larger purpose. Just like every one of us, you are a gift to the world. And there is no way you can serve in the capacity that you are called to serve if you are sick.

Mission Is Purpose

We challenge you to realize that you have a vital purpose on this planet. We are convinced that the world will never be what it could be—what it should be—until everyone steps up to fulfill his or her purpose. The foundation is good health. If you aren't healthy, you won't be able to step up.

Please reread the paragraph above and let it sink in. Then reread this section a couple of times before you go forward. Because if you don't get this, you won't be able to transform. You have to understand your "why." And so for us, mission is purpose.

Savor the Fringe Benefits

Then and only then are there all those other benefits. You look better, you feel better. You even smell better! You can jump higher. You can engage in sports longer. You can be sixty-seven years old and not need a nap just because you played with your grandkids. You get to enjoy life. That's the biggest fringe benefit of all. These gifts are the natural consequences, the healthy and positive side effects of finding and living your why.

We've told you our whys in our tales of transformation. Once again, we challenge you to come up with your "whys." Write them down in your Transformation Journal and review them regularly, particularly if and when you are finding it hard to stay the course.

Welcome to a New Lifestyle

In the following pages, you'll learn how to use essential oils and certain foods as aids to help you reach your ideal weight and prevent chronic disease. Understand that quick fixes, which are typically short-lived, are not what this book is about. That said, we can all but guarantee that you will see transformational results after just a single week on our program. In fact, we have no doubt that you will be so impressed that you will be inspired to permanently change your lifestyle, resulting in vibrant health, a longer lifespan, a slimmer body, and a belief in the power of your commitment. Losing excess pounds—and keeping them off this time—is just one of many joyful changes you will experience!

To help you along the journey, we have created a series of demo videos on food prep and food shopping, preparing essential oil remedies, exercise, and more. Each of the videos contains extra insights into the strategies and information covered in this book. You can access these videos free at EssentialOilsDiet.com.

PART 1

THE PROBLEM AND THE SOLUTION

CHAPTER 1

WHY "DIETS" FAIL BUT TRANSFORMATION WORKS

"Therefore, I urge you, brothers and sisters, in view of God's mercy, to offer your bodies as a living sacrifice, holy and pleasing to God—this is your true and proper worship. Do not conform to the pattern of this world but be transformed by the renewing of your mind. Then you will be able to test and approve what God's will is—His good, pleasing and perfect will."

—ROMANS 12:1–2

Are you impatient to get to the recipes and guidelines for the Essential Oils Diet? Are you eager to start using essential oils to support your weight loss? Are you hoping that this combination of food and essential oils may be the magic bullet that finally allows you to take control of your eating habits?

Whoa! Let's slow down for a moment. Jumping in too quickly without understanding the strategy behind our program could all too soon turn your enthusiasm to disappointment. Our recipes are delicious, easy to prepare, and nutritious, and the use of essential oils to assist in weight loss is backed by solid research. We even have an exercise program that you can quickly incorporate into your daily routine. Our approach is flexible enough to fit any lifestyle and food preferences. And we are excited to share our wonderful essential oil blends to moderate hunger, salves to help massage away belly fat, and the exercises Sabrina has designed to tone your body.

All well and good, but without a firm mind-set transformed to focus on success, a commitment to make these new habits a way of life, and a belief in the outcome of your actions, you may wind up a few months from now discouraged and searching for yet another magic bullet to banish your extra pounds.

That is the last thing we want you to experience. Instead, we want to encourage you to embark on a transformative journey.

So, slow down and let us explain the underlying principles that ground the Essential Oils Diet. Trust us, doing so will significantly increase your likelihood of succeeding on the program. In fact, the changes we are talking about are nothing less than transformational. Both of us have experienced such dramatic and lasting changes in our own lives, which we shared in the introduction. Our hope and our belief is that this book will provide the blessings of such an experience to all who read it and commit to our program.

If you're a page skimmer or simply skipped the preface and/or introduction, we urge you to go back and pay special attention to that *essential* content. You will get so much more out of this book—and we're not just talking about taking control of your weight, we're talking about changing your life—if you understand where we are coming from *and* follow the steps we have laid out.

Two Sides of the Same Coin

At its core, this is a healthy living book. Live a healthy life and you're going to lose weight just by virtue of being healthy. And as part of this commitment to health, you'll learn ways to accelerate weight loss. For example, we'll explain how matcha green tea contains fat-burning compounds called catechins. Another example: You'll learn how simply inhaling lime essential oil can help burn body fat.

We understand that initially the goal of transformation to good health is rather abstract, while seeing excess pounds melt away is a more immediate and exciting transformation. Fortunately, the Essential Oils Diet achieves both goals.

The Truth About Diets

We hate to break it to you, but weight-loss diets almost always fail, but *not* because you cannot stick with a certain program, have a genetic tendency to be overweight, have a burdened metabolism, or suffer from a damaged microbiome. We know that this statement flies in the face of what you have read elsewhere. Some of these supposed causes are myths, others apply to very few people, and still others are a result, not a cause, of weight gain.

As we alerted you in the preface, this is not a conventional diet book. By that we mean food is not at the core of the problem—nor is it the solution. If you follow the Essential Oils Diet, we can all but promise that you will find your body's ideal weight. Most people will lose weight. If you need to lose a lot of weight, you will do so relatively quickly. We know that obesity is directly linked to the development of cancer, diabetes, and autoimmune disorders, so once you begin your transformation, you won't be as susceptible to these diseases. Bonus!

The Essential Oils Diet is a two-stage program. As the name implies, the Essential Fast Track helps you banish excess pounds quickly— think readying for your daughter's wedding, a Caribbean vacation, or a college reunion—but more importantly, it is the gateway to the Essential Lifestyle. The startup lasts for thirty days, or longer if you have more than ten pounds to banish.

Now let's take a good, hard look at why most if not all weight-loss diets fail.

Useless and Misleading Information

The Nutrition Facts panel on food labels is of no real help in telling you whether a food item is worth eating. Do you really know what constitutes a gram of sugar, fiber, or carbohydrate, other than the fact that it is a tiny amount? And does looking at the numbers of grams and percentages of calories and fats really tell you whether something benefits your health or will help you control your weight? Of course not.

The only part of packaged food labels that is remotely helpful is the ingredients list, although that usually just alerts you to the fact that there are numerous ingredients you've neither heard of nor can pronounce because you don't have a degree in toxicology!

In 1980, the US Department of Health and Human Services and the US Department of Agriculture (USDA) jointly released *Nutrition and Your Health: Dietary Guidelines for Americans* in an effort to educate the public about how to eat. The food pyramid was designed to be a visual representation of the dietary guidelines, but it was equally incomprehensible, which is undoubtedly why it was laid to rest a few years ago and replaced with a graphic called MyPlate. This is equally unhelpful in determining what to eat and how much of it. But here's the kicker: Guess when the rise in overweight and obesity began? You guessed it— 1980. And it has continued to climb stratospherically ever since.[1]

The food pyramid was incorrect, and nutrition labels remain useless because they focus only on "essential" nutrients, meaning such things as protein, carbs, vitamins, and minerals your body cannot make on its own but are essential for life. Neither the food pyramid nor nutrition labels focus on so-called nonessential nutrients such as bioactive compounds, which provide an abundant life of vibrant health. Yes, essential nutrients are necessary to keep you alive. You could stay alive on a feeding tube, but it wouldn't mean you're truly alive. More on this distinction in chapter 2.

A food label provides only a bare minimum of information. A

minimalist attitude connotes just squeaking by. What's the least I can do? Diets fail because their approach encourages the human tendency to do the bare minimum, not to go above and beyond. Diets don't offer an abundant mind-set. It's like "What's the lowest possible grade I could get on this test to pass the class?" The fact that we're still talking only about vitamins and minerals and protein and carbs just shows us that, as a society, our understanding of nutrition is archaic.

Most egregious of all, the recommended daily value (RDV) percentages that you see on food labels are based on a 2,000-calorie-a-day diet. First off, most people do not even realize this. Secondly, even if they did, they wouldn't know how to make this knowledge even the slightest bit useful!

Case in point: Do you know how many calories you should be eating each day? How about your spouse? Your youngest child? Your teenager? Do you know how much they should be consuming? If you did, would this change the foods you served your family?

Truth is, you have no idea and neither do we, because no one knows! It's literally impossible to calculate your caloric needs on a daily basis. And making your food choices on RDVs should not—we repeat *should not*—determine your food choices.

To watch a video shopping tour in which we show you how we read food labels and choose the best foods in supermarkets, go to EssentialOilsDiet.com.

The number of calories required to sustain a healthy, abundant life depends on your age, weight, height, metabolic type, activity level, and a slew of other factors that would make your head spin if we listed them all. Suffice it to say that your caloric needs on any given day will definitely not be the same on any other given day. Not to mention that the same applies to each member of your family!

To base your daily intake of vitamins, minerals, and macronutrients (carbs, proteins, and fats) on the percentages listed on your food labels is utterly illogical. This count-by-numbers approach has dominated the field of nutrition for decades, replacing common sense.

Diets Are Unsustainable

Another reason so many diets don't work in the long term is that they are unrealistically restrictive. Their focus is on short-term abstinence for quick weight loss, not long-term transformation.

If you have followed a low-carb diet that eliminated or drastically cut down on fruit, grains, and other carbohydrate-rich foods, you probably saw some pounds fall away. Low-fat diets tell you to eliminate or drastically reduce fat intake. Ketogenic diets advise just the opposite: eat lots of fat. Paleo diets are typically fat and protein heavy. This conflicting information is enough to give you a severe case of diet whiplash!

Cutting out almost all fat or carbohydrates is just plain unrealistic for the vast majority of people. (Nor is it healthy or natural to *overeat* protein and/or fat.) When you follow a rigid program, you may be missing out on important micronutrients essential to good health. And after a while, even if you can stick with such a restrictive program, your body adapts to it and weight loss ceases.

The bottom line is, if a way of eating isn't satisfying and enjoyable, you're more than likely going to revert to what you've enjoyed in the past. (And if you are the main cook in the family, preparing one meal for yourself and another for the rest of the gang gets old fast.) That's why most "diets" work for a few weeks or a few months, until a person is impelled to "cheat," gets discouraged, and goes back to her old way of eating, with predictable results.

We cannot stress enough how flexible our program is. If you have certain food sensitivities or allergies, simply avoid those foods. If you're a vegan or a vegetarian, no problem—in fact, this is a plant-centric program. If you hate such and such a food, no one is saying you have to eat it. When it comes to essential oils, each person's response to a specific oil is different, and we'll help you find the ones that work best for you.

Unless a diet becomes a lifestyle, as you'll learn that the Essential Oils Diet does, it is almost invariably doomed to failure.

BEWARE OF THE YO-YO EFFECT

All too often people regain all the lost weight or even add on a few extra pounds when they return to their "normal" diet. This is referred to as the "yo-yo effect," and it happens a lot with low-carb, high-fat diets.

Of all the various food plans out there, the yo-yo effect is most profound in the ketogenic diet—an approach similar to the Atkins diet in that it heavily restricts the consumption of fruits, grains, and legumes, with the result that 5 percent of your energy intake comes from carbs, 15 to 25 percent from protein, and about 75 percent from fat. It's important to realize that a vast majority of research trials evaluating keto's effect on humans have lasted only a few weeks or a couple of months at most. There is no way to determine the long-term weight-loss benefits from current studies. Animal studies, however, are more robust and suggest that the weight loss achieved is relatively short-lived.

Longer-term animal studies reveal that weight loss ceases after eighteen to twenty-two weeks on the ketogenic diet, at which point weight starts to return to normal and then gradually increases[2, 3]. This is not to say that humans will gain weight after following a keto approach for five or six months; we're simply pointing out that the literature does not support long-term benefits for people following ketogenic and other low-carb diets, and it also suggests that the weight-loss benefits will be relatively short-lived.

The Absence of Abundance

The Healing Power of Essential Oils was all about helping you use essential oils to enjoy an abundant life. Another reason why diets fail and why transformation works is because the restriction inherent in diets completely ignores the concept of abundance. We can deny ourselves satisfying, tasty food for only so long. There are numerous ways the Essential Oils Diet enables you to have your cake and eat it, too, including a recipe for the healthy, naturally sweetened, abundant-life-giving Our Carrot Wedding Cake (page 270).

Denial is unsustainable. No one in her right mind wants to remain in boot camp the rest of her life. We know that the Essential Fast Track isn't sustainable for a long period of time, just as a low-fat or low-carb diet isn't. No strict program is satisfying long-term. Instead, the Essential Fast Track morphs into a natural and abundant way of eating you can enjoy for the rest of your life.

Time Is of the Essence

All too many diets boast that you can lose ten, twenty, thirty, or some impressive number of pounds in as many days. This is completely unrealistic and sets you up for failure. Initial weight loss almost always slows over time. Conceivably, someone who is extremely overweight and restricts her intake dramatically for a month could lose thirty pounds, but that is hardly the norm. That's why most thirty-day diets fail. It is simply not enough time to take off weight and maintain that loss when the person returns to her old way of eating. You need to continue beyond thirty days, which is why we have you transition into the Essential Lifestyle, which is designed to be a permanent way of eating, after the Essential Fast Track.

No More Cheat Days

Another reason that diets don't work is that many of them allow a cheat day. If you are eating tasty, satisfying food, there is no need for days off. In direct contrast, the Essential Oils Diet includes a fasting day once a week in the program's second phase. A day—or partial day, if you prefer—of fasting has been shown to enhance not just weight control but a number of other health benefits. You'll learn more about the multiple benefits of fasting in Part 2.

"Slow" Metabolism Is Not a Scapegoat

The final reason why diets fail is that most are largely focused on the wrong thing: boosting your metabolism so you can burn fat as though it's as simple as adding some high-octane fuel to your car to optimize performance.

The word *metabolism* derives from the Greek word for change, meaning the whole range of biochemical transformations within an organism's cells that are required for life. In plain English, your metabolism influences your body's basic energy needs.

Contrary to popular belief, there's little evidence to support the claim that weight gain is linked to a slow metabolism. Well, at least according to major government health agencies and hospitals such as the Mayo Clinic and the United Kingdom's National Health Services (NHS).

Yes, it's true that your metabolism and body weight are connected, but as the Mayo Clinic points out, "Metabolism is rarely the cause of excess weight gain. . . . How much you eat and drink along with how much physical activity you get are the things that ultimately determine your weight."[4]

We are not exactly sure how this myth started and how a slow metabolism became the scapegoat for those troublesome extra pounds and expanding waistlines. This is particularly strange because the NHS clearly states that "research actually shows that overweight people have faster metabolisms than thinner people. Larger bodies require more energy to carry out basic bodily functions."[5]

The problem here is also one of accountability. We have discovered that blaming weight gain on one's "metabolism" allows people to feel that they are not accountable for their actions. In fact, every single day too many people burden their metabolism by eating chemical-laden processed foods and introducing other toxins via equally chemical-laden body care products and pharmaceutical and recreational drugs, among other factors.

Instead of maintaining the very metabolic processes that keep us alive, this kind of behavior forces the body to expend vital energy eliminating these toxins. The result is that the monopolized metabolism cannot properly digest and assimilate foods and the normal function of fat-burning for energy becomes a second priority, compromising the body's ability to find an ideal weight and fight disease. Negative thoughts and stress aggravate the situation. Essentially, many people are barely surviving, much less thriving.

On the other hand, the bioactive compounds in the foods you'll be eating on our program can help your body reset its metabolism, which will help you get healthy and find your body's natural weight.

The Real Deal

In almost all cases, the real cause of being overweight is twofold: poor food choices and overeating because the food consumed fails to satisfy. But before you beat yourself up, understand that this is not all your fault, as we'll discuss in chapter 3. Once you alter your way of eating and make some other lifestyle changes, you will discover the amazing power of transformation that eliminates those unhealthy cravings.

Stick with the Essential Fast Track and you will experience that "aha" moment that is the gateway to freedom from your addiction to the unhealthy foods. (As research clearly has pointed out, sugar is more addictive than cocaine.[6]) We'll explore the difference between self-control and faith that something is working. Once that aha moment occurs, you'll never be tempted again. (Or, if temptation does rear its ugly head, you can rest assured that you have the tools to have that internal dialogue with yourself—and God.) It's important to understand that transformation is different for each one of us. Nor does it necessarily happen in one fell swoop as it did for Dr. Z. For Mama Z, a progression of steps moved her inevitably toward transformation.

Changing Old Habits, Making New Habits

A recent study divided overweight individuals into three groups. In addition to following a standard weight-loss program, one group of participants was instructed to follow ten habit-forming tips, such as improving awareness of food intake, for twelve weeks; another group was told to exercise differently or break an old daily habit—which did not need to be health related—such as always driving to work the same way; the third (the control group) was told to simply follow their normal daily routine and were given no weight-loss advice. When the researchers followed up with the subjects after twelve weeks, the first two groups had lost significantly more weight than the control group (6.8 pounds on average). After twelve months, both these groups maintained an average weight loss of 5 percent of their original weight. They had demonstrated that forming new habits and breaking old habits, indicating an openness to change, enabled those subjects to maintain their weight loss.[7]

Don't be discouraged; this isn't to say that it will take twelve weeks for you to form a new habit. But it definitely takes some time!

Much has been written about forming habits, much of it contradictory, with the magic number ranging anywhere from twenty-one days to more than a year. Phillippa Lally, a psychology researcher at University College London, and her associates examined the habits of ninety-six individuals over a twelve-week period. Each subject was asked to choose a single new habit and report daily on whether he had complied and how automatic it was to perform the new habit. The researchers found that it takes an average of 66 days for a habit to become automatic, but some people were able to form a new habit in as little as 18 days, while others took as long as 254 days.[8]

Obviously, different people tackling different habits of differing complexity accounted in large part for the variation. Knowing this, we have streamlined the transition from the thirty-day Essential Fast Track plan to the Essential Lifestyle phase by minimizing the food variations. Nor are there any new diet restrictions that you'll need to implement. In fact, quite the opposite.

Honing Habits

There are more options to choose from and more foods to eat in the Essential Lifestyle, which will empower you to continue for many years to come. The transformations we will walk you through in phase 2 are more lifestyle-oriented in nature, making them easy to implement because you will already be familiar with the food modifications!

Believe us, once you begin to practice certain behaviors in the Essential Fast Track, they will slowly become habitual. But we're not going to kid you. There will be challenges in the first month. It will take some time, some effort, some strategizing to get through it. And you're not done after that first month. Remember, it takes more than twenty-one days on average to establish new habits. But if you continue and are faithful to the program and your new habits, you're setting yourself up to sustain a healthier lifestyle for the long term.

The Beginning of Transformation

Once you have reformed your poor eating habits, something surprising happens. You find yourself thinking, "Wow! I simply have no desire to eat this food anymore." That desire has been removed from your heart—and therefore your body doesn't crave it.

To us, a habit is synonymous with transformation. By virtue of forming a new habit, you have been transformed. You could say that habit is the physical manifestation of an internal transformation.

More specifically, habits are a physical manifestation of a spiritual transformation. Transformation has to happen in your spirit before it becomes ingrained, or natural, so to speak. It has to happen in your heart, in your mind, in your soul before you start to live it out: "Without even thinking about it, this is the way I do such and such." So a habit is proof that you have been transformed.

Dreams take root in the heart. Whatever your objectives and personal beliefs, we urge you to regard your experience with the Essential Oils Diet as a kind of spiritual journey. Hold yourself accountable. You can also serve others by example, or better yet if your success makes you want to share the good news with family, friends, and your community. Newly ingrained habits transform you. And those around you will notice that transformation, which can lead to *their* transformation.

Three Steps Forward, Two Steps Back

While you are in the process of changing your habits, don't despair if you occasionally fall back or forget to consistently practice a new behavior. Importantly, don't use an occasional lapse as a reason to go back to your old lifestyle. Such missteps are actually learning opportunities.

Dr. Z here. I'm grateful for all the times I've fallen down. Like the book of Proverbs says, "The righteous person will fall seven times yet get up again." As your habits become automatic, you will be transformed. And I'm always encouraged by Proverbs 4:18, which is my life verse: "The path of the righteous is like the rising of the dawn that gets brighter and brighter to the full light of day."

The Caterpillar and the Butterfly

Think of transformation as metamorphosis, like going from a caterpillar to a butterfly. You are still the same person but dramatically changed, or reborn with a fresh set of eyes. If someone is unwilling to dive in, to give it her all, she can never really change and therefore cannot be completely transformed. She is wasting her time. That's why the idea of a cheat day, which is part of many weight-loss programs, is simply not in our vocabulary. There's no way that either of us is going to go back to doing what we were doing.

The caterpillar is also a metaphor for the two phases of our program. Think of the thirty-day Fast Track as the time the caterpillar spends morphing in the cocoon she has woven for herself. Your thirty-day walk with us—like a caterpillar hunkering down for lifelong transformation—could be lonely and scary. You may want to isolate yourself from people who will try to influence you in a bad way. Your reward will be the emergence into the Essential Lifestyle as the beautiful butterfly that sheds her cocoon, opens her wings, and flies free.

We want to encourage other people to open themselves up to transformation, and we believe the Essential Fast Track provides the path. We can give you all the tools to follow the program in the following chapters, but we can't tell you exactly how to transform. It is different for everyone. But if you are starting to identify the unhealthy behaviors you're engaging in that need to change, you are on the right track.

We're going to end this chapter with a bit of tough love: If you do not take the time to follow the basics of the Essential Oils Diet, you're not going to get anything out of this book. But if you do, we can promise your life will be transformed.

CHAPTER 2

THE ANTIDOTE TO CHEMICAL SOUP: BIOACTIVE-RICH FOODS AND ESSENTIAL OILS

"One cannot think well, love well, sleep well, if one has not dined well."
—VIRGINIA WOOLF

To our knowledge, the Essential Oils Diet is the first program that integrates essential oils and bioactive-rich foods, demonstrating how they can work in tandem to help you achieve a healthy weight and prevent disease.

In this chapter, we'll explain what bioactive compounds are and cover the basics of aromatherapy. Then in Part 2, you'll learn how food can work synergistically with essential oils to help you reach your health goals, and we'll outline exactly what you need to do. But first, we need to address why it's important that we incorporate bioactive compounds into your lifestyle.

The "Chemical Soup" in Food, Air, and Everywhere

Every day you are exposed to a cocktail of chemicals that interact with each other in ways that are far beyond human understanding. You must be vigilant to minimize your consumption of this "chemical soup," as we refer to it. You are undoubtedly aware that nonorganic food is regularly sprayed with toxic pesticides, herbicides, and fungicides, but this is just the beginning of how much our food is tainted.

Did you know that "baby carrots" are made from deformed carrots that failed to meet grocery store appearance requirements? An extensive manufacturing process shapes them into the cocktail carrots that are often served with dips—or fed to kids. Because their protective skin has been peeled off, these carrots will oxidize, which tints them white. To keep them bright orange, they are dipped in or sprayed with chlorine—yes, the same stuff used to bleach clothes. This, despite the fact that chlorine is a well-known carcinogen, which has been shown to cause liver malfunction, deplete your immune system, and set the stage for atherosclerosis.[1,2,3] Swimming in a chlorinated pool puts people at higher risks of developing asthma, thanks to dangerous aromatic compounds of chlorine gas.[4]

Because most chemicals in our food are still relatively new, we are flying blind when it comes to their long-term health effects. However, research suggests that these effects may persist throughout life and may even be deadly. For example, according to the work produced by the Greater Boston Physicians for Social Responsibility entitled *In Harm's Way: Toxic Threats to Child Development*,[5] millions of American children already suffer from numerous neurocognitive disorders due to chemical exposure in their food and environment, including learning disabilities (e.g., ADD, ADHD, autism), reduced IQ, destructive and aggressive behavior, and some social disorders.

Organophosphates (insecticides such as diazinon) and other pesticides widely used in homes and schools accumulate in the food chain, and ultimately in your body's tissues, and are among the most dangerous. These chemicals literally prevent proper hormone and cellular function and disrupt the flow of neurotransmitters or other growth factors.[6] Nonetheless, these toxins are regularly used in food manufacturing and pollute our environment. A pregnant woman passes them on to her unborn child via the placenta and later through breast milk. When we eat foods that contain these poisons, they take up permanent residence in our bones, blood, fat, urine, ovaries, and sperm.

Organic farmers use Citrox, a nontoxic citrus-based solution, to preserve baby carrots, rather than chlorine as in conventionally raised carrots. Better yet, slice up regular carrots into spears.

Ambushed by Antibiotics

Another major group of ingredients in chemical soup is antibiotics. Fully half of prescribed antibiotics are not needed or are ineffective as prescribed.[7] Antibiotics are also fed to cows, chickens, and other animals, including farmed fish, to prevent disease in crowded quarters and promote growth.[8] If you eat conventional meat and dairy or farmed fish, these drugs wind up in your body. Overuse leads to antibiotic resistance, making the drugs less effective or ineffective, which can have dire implications. Every year more than 23,000 Americans die because of antibiotic-resistant infections.[9] One such condition is *Clostridium difficile* (aka *C. diff*), which sends 250,000 people to the hospital annually, of whom 14,000 don't survive.

The easiest way to understand how antibiotics work in your body is to compare them to ordering a nuclear attack when sending a sharpshooter would do the job. This broad-spectrum approach does considerable damage to your entire immune system. Recent studies have suggested that antibiotic use encourages the growth of the yeast *Candida albicans,* which opens your body to a slew of health issues,[10] such as the following:

- Chronic fatigue
- Brain fog
- Foul body odor
- Insomnia
- Low libido
- Sugar cravings
- Seasonal allergies

Eighty percent of your immune system lies in your gut,[11] so any attack on healthy bacteria puts your body at risk. One common effect antibiotics have on the delicate microfloral balance is leaky gut syndrome and related skin problems like acne or rosacea. They have also been shown to cause various food allergies and other autoimmune disorders, as well as tendon rupture.[12] Some responses are even more dire, including kidney failure, psychotic reactions, retinal detachment, neurotoxicity, and disruptions in blood sugar metabolism.[13] With four out of five Americans taking an antibiotic each year, we are at risk for a public health pandemic!

Beyond Vitamins and Minerals

We are big proponents of what we call an abundant lifestyle with a holistic approach to health. What you consume and breathe, the products you put on your body and use in your home, the water you drink, and proper supplementation, plus regular movement and exercise, are all essential to mental and physical health. Also crucial is removing toxins from your body on a regular basis, through both fasting and bowel cleansing. All these factors above are also essential to optimal health, but the foundation upon which the Essential Oils Diet is built is bioactive-rich foods and essential oils—which are themselves bioactive.

Unless you are a food scientist, you may be scratching your head and wondering, "What exactly does the word *bioactive* mean? And why haven't I heard of it?" Not to worry. When we ran the word by a bunch of colleagues in the natural health field, they were not familiar with it either.

Although it sounds similar, bioactive is not the same as *biodynamic,* which refers to a way of organic farming developed by the twentieth-century Austrian philosopher and social reformer Rudolf Steiner. Nor should it be confused with *bioavailability,* which refers to the rate and degree at which the body can use nutrients or medications.

ANTIBIOTIC AVOIDANCE

You can avoid or at least minimize the double onslaught of pesticides in food and overuse of antibiotics.

- *Avoid antibiotics as much as possible.* If you are prescribed a fluoride-containing fluoroquinolone antibiotic such as Cipro, Levaquin, Avelox, ciprofloxacin, levofloxacin, or moxifloxacin, ask if it is absolutely necessary.

- *Use essential oils more.* Oregano oil has been proven to be more effective than conventional antibiotics in clinical trials.[14] It also has powerful antifungal properties, so you don't have to worry about candida overgrowth as you would with antibiotics.

- *Don't get sick in the first place!* Easier said than done, right? But the Essential Oils Diet is full of bioactive compounds that will enable you to fight off the common cold and flu. It will be the beginning of an empowering realization that you are in control of your health!

- *Consume probiotics.* Enhance your immune function by regularly consuming probiotic-rich foods such as coconut yogurt and kimchi. Be sure to load up on raw, multi-strain probiotic supplements during cold and flu season. We like the Garden of Life brand.

Let us explain. Surely you've heard of fiber. Well, guess what? Fiber is a bioactive compound. Surely you've heard of antioxidants. Maybe you've heard of polyphenols. Well, all of these are bioactive compounds.

Bioactive compounds are defined as the "components of food that influence physiological or cellular activities in the animals or humans that consume them."[15] Specifically, they are "phytochemicals found in foods that are capable of modulating metabolic processes and resulting in the promotion of better health."[16]

The flavors and colors that make vegetables and fruit appealing and stimulate our senses are the result of bioactive compounds. They are also found in some animal foods, namely cold-water fish such as salmon, which boast bioactive compounds in the form of essential fatty acids.

The bottom line is the plant foods we eat and the herbal remedies we use—including essential oils—contain bioactive compounds. Some are more robust than others, however, and that's the focus of the Essential Oils Diet: to consume bioactive-rich foods and essential oils to shed excess pounds and achieve abundant health! The focus of our approach is to bolster our so-called nonessential nutrition and not concentrate on simply consuming the bare minimums to meet the baseless recommended daily values of fats, proteins, and carbs. We're going way beyond vitamins and minerals here!

Truly Essential Nutrition

Let us explain in greater detail why some nutrients are classified as "essential" and others as "nonessential." The terms are understandably confusing. Essential nutrients are those that are required for life that cannot be made on their own, and therefore they must be provided by your diet. Think carbohydrates, protein, fat, vitamins, minerals, and water. Like essential nutrients, nonessential nutrients are still required for human life, but the body *can* make them on its own. Examples include certain amino acids, cholesterol, fiber, and vitamin D. These nonessential nutrients are also the bioactive substances found in food.[17]

There are other nonnutritive bioactive compounds found in food that are technically not required for survival, but without their regular consumption, our lives would be much less pleasant. You know and love these compounds as essential oils.

The Benefits of Bioactives

Scientists engaged in cutting-edge research are finally putting a name to something we hadn't qualified until now. Think of it this way: bioactive compounds are like the pen pal you felt you knew but now are meeting face-to-face. To our knowledge, this is the first book that makes sense of the role bioactive-rich foods play in living a healthy life and controlling your weight.

Basically, your health is either robust or poor, depending on your diet's proportion of bioactive-rich foods. Many of these compounds are present in foods that you are probably already eating, but we will help you make them a more essential component of your diet.

Bioactives such as flavonoids, carotenoids, and polyphenols are all plant chemicals with antioxidant properties that protect your body's cells from damage caused by unstable atoms called free radicals, which cause illness and hasten aging. If your diet is lacking in an array of foods full of different bioactive compounds, you're going to be sick—and you're going to gain weight.

There are thousands of bioactive compounds: more than eight thousand polyphenols alone have been identified to date! A diet replete with bioactive compounds fine-tunes your metabolism so your energy level remains high throughout the day, enabling both mental and physical peak performance.

Such a diet also enables you to burn calories efficiently, keeping your weight under control. In particular, plant-based foods contain a complex mix of many of these compounds that act in an integrative manner, which is why real food is always a better nutrition source than a single vitamin supplement, multivitamin, or powder mix. We're going to show you how to incorporate more bioactive compounds into your meals with whole foods, herbs, and essential oils. And once you familiarize yourself wth Mama Z's recipes, you'll also understand how to "remodel" your own favorite recipes to make them more bioactive rich.

The Essence of Bioactivity

Bioactive compounds have the ability to communicate with your body's tissues on a cellular level, impacting the metabolic processes that keep it running like a well-oiled machine.[18] Check out the Essential Eight (page 78) for more detail on some of the most important bioactive-rich foods you'll be eating and how they impact your health and your weight.

Dr. Z here. Scientists refer to bioactive compounds as "extra-nutritional," meaning they contain no calories (as protein, fat, and carbohydrates do), and they are not vitamins or minerals. Nor, as we just discussed, are they considered essential nutrients. But this does not make them any less significant healthwise. Without bioactive compounds in your meals, you could still be alive but would be one sick puppy!

Bioactive components occur in small amounts in foods, but their effects can have a large impact. Numerous epidemiologic studies have shown that a plant-based diet rich in bioactive nutrients can help prevent cardiovascular disease and cancer.[19] (Epidemiology is a field of medicine that studies the incidence of disease in certain populations.)

In addition to flavonoids and carotenoids, bioactive compounds include phytoestrogens (plant estrogens) found in flaxseed oil. Several compounds act as antioxidants, including resveratrol, present in nuts and red wine, and lycopene, found in tomatoes. Bioactive compounds in onions, scallions, leeks, garlic, cruciferous vegetables such as cabbage and cauliflower, many citrus fruits, cherries, and herbs also appear to protect against cancer and heart disease.

The Next Big Thing in the Food Industry?

Although the word *bioactive* may be still under the radar for most people, its significance is not lost on food manufacturers. You can bet that scientists in their employ are already figuring out how to use carotenoids, essential oils, antioxidants, and other bioactive compounds in new packaged foods made with added flavors "in order to enhance their sensory properties or to develop their nutritional and health properties."[22] Ditto for supplement makers eager to jump on the bioactive-compounds bandwagon. This means the next great marketing term following *natural*—which is meaningless—*organic, non-GMO,* and *gluten free* may well be *bioactive*!

TOO MUCH MEAT!

Research has shown that diets low in bioactive compounds will ultimately lead to subpar health. This is particularly important in light of the recent spike in interest surrounding carbohydrate-starvation fad diets that promote heavy consumption of meat and animal fat.

Now, we're not saying that people will get sick and die young if they regularly eat meat, though studies have alluded to this as a possibility, with an increased risk of heart disease as one major threat.[20] We're simply pointing out that research strongly suggests that someone's chance of enjoying optimal health is greatly diminished if her diet consists primarily of animal fat and protein. The reason? These low-carb fad diets focus on "essential nutrition" and ignore bioactive compounds, which are responsible for robust health.

The *European Journal of Nutrition* published an article in 2013 that put it this way: "Whereas the absence of essential nutrients from the diet results in overt deficiency often times with moderate to severe physiological decrements, the absence of bioactive substances from the diet results in suboptimal health."[21]

Which would you choose? Enjoy "suboptimal health" to shed some quick pounds or follow our approach, which will help you reach your ideal weight and enjoy long-lasting health for years to come?

Rather than spending your hard-earned dollars on supplements containing these compounds, your new way of eating organically grown, non-GMO fruits, vegetables, ancient whole grains (oatmeal, quinoa, millet, brown rice, spelt, amaranth, sorghum, and teff), legumes, healthy fats, and nuts will offer the countless health benefits found in bioactive-rich foods. Mama Z's recipes in Part 3 (page 203) are packed with bioactives.

The Bioactive Compounds
Known as Essential Oils

Millions of people already use essential oils for health, well-being, and relaxation. You may be among them, particularly if you have already read Dr. Z's first book, *The Healing Power of Essential Oils*. Essential oils are inherently bioactive, but unlike bioactive-rich foods, essential oils are not a source of nutrition. For example, both the fruit of the lemon and lemon essential oil (extracted from the rind) contain bioactive compounds, but the latter doesn't provide any energy in the form of calories, vitamins, or minerals. However, together they become far more than the sum of their parts.

While foods supply energy in the form of calories and many contain small amounts of bioactive compounds, essential oils offer a more concentrated form of bioactivity. In fact, they symbolize the essence of bioactivity—minute but highly concentrated compounds able to heal body (and soul) with metabolic effects that can assist in weight loss—or weight gain if that is your concern. Certain oils can also boost your energy level, so you can be more active and burn more body fat.

In chapter 6, we'll show you exactly how to use essential oils to reach your goal weight and prevent chronic disease. But, before we do, let's give you a primer on aromatherapy.

The Essence of Nature

"And the leaves of the tree are for the healing of the nations" *(Revelations 22:2)*. We can think of no other substance on earth that epitomizes this Bible verse better than essential oils. Extracted directly from the bark, flowers, leaves, resins, and roots of plants, essential oils are highly concentrated plant-based chemical compounds recognized for thousands of years for their healing prowess. When you realize that it takes three hundred pounds of rose petals, sixty pounds of lavender, or up to forty-five pounds of lemon rinds to fill a single fifteen-milliliter bottle with essential oil, you appreciate how extraordinarily concentrated they are. They are bioactives in their purest form!

As you can tell, it takes vastly different amounts of the various plant compounds to fill that itty-bitty container, which is one reason why the prices of various oils differ considerably. Another mind-boggling fact is that just one drop of essential oil contains up to three hundred powerfully life-changing chemicals naturally found in plants that serve to resist disease, attract bees and other pollinators, and protect plants from predators.

It may surprise you to learn two things about essential oils. First, essential oils are not "essential." And, second, they are not "oils."

The scientific term for essential oils is *volatile organic compound,* which paints a much better picture of what we're referring to. The volatile components of a plant are the parts that are released quickly into the air. The *Encyclopedia Britannica* describes the naming rationale this way: "Essential oil, highly volatile substance isolated by a physical process from an odoriferous plant of a single botanical species. . . . Such oils were called essential because they were thought to represent the very essence of odour and flavour."[23]

The essential oil is why you smell lavender when you lean down and sniff the blooms. It releases as you walk through the garden and brush against the plants. The scientists who had the privilege of naming this chemical component believed the oils to be "essential" to the plant as much as they were volatile (quickly released).

Essential oils also are not oils, which are the liquid form of fats (i.e., lipids) at room temperature. Like lipids, essential oils are insoluble in water; hence the misnomer "essential oil." However, because the components of essential oils are terpenes, they differ from fatty oils because they do not contain the glycerides of fatty acids.[24]

Rather, they are the lipophilic (i.e., fat-loving) and hydrophobic (i.e., water-hating) volatile organic compounds found in plants. In practical terms, this means essential oils dissolve readily in fat but don't mix easily with water. This characteristic of essential oils is also one reason why they are transdermal, which means they literally penetrate your skin, making their way into your bloodstream and into the cells throughout your body within minutes of application. This is the reason why they leave no residue after you apply them to your skin.

Using Essential Oils Is as Easy as 1-2-3

There are three basic ways to use essential oils: inhale them, apply them on your skin, or consume them. All three come into play in the Essential Oils Diet, so let's briefly look at each approach.

To watch a free screening of our ten-part video master class on how to use essential oils, visit EssentialOilsForAbundantLiving.com.

INHALATION

Considered the safest and most popular aromatherapy method, the use of a diffuser—specifically, an ultrasonic steam diffuser—is a great way to start your essential oils practice. These diffusers contain a vibrating disc beneath a water reservoir that breaks up the volatile organic compounds into countless microparticles and disperses them via a fine mist. (Alternatively, you can get the aromatic benefits of essential oils by placing several drops in a pot of water and bringing it to a simmer on the cooktop.)

There are few risks to using a diffuser, even around children and pets. To use your diffuser, simply follow these steps:

- Fill it with purified or distilled water up to the "fill line" or "fill marker."
- Check the water capacity and add 4 or 5 drops of essential oil for each 100 to 150 milliliters of water. With essential oils, a little goes a long way.

That's pretty easy, isn't it? Unless you prefer to do so, there's no need to keep the diffuser running all the time. The benefits continue even after diffusion has ceased.

Safety First: Make sure that the room in which you use a diffuser is well ventilated, particularly if there are children or pets in the household. When you first start to diffuse essential oils, run the diffuser for only a few minutes to gauge your reaction. Likewise, when you use a new scent or new blend, take it slow. Assuming you don't get a headache, experience sinus issues, or have another adverse reaction, slowly but surely increase the amount of time you run the diffuser, up to several hours.

A DIFFUSER IS ESSENTIAL

If you have any doubt that essential oils are wildly popular, take a look at the number of diffusers on the market. They come in a variety of materials, designs, and colors, but the features you want to focus on are capacity, ease of operation, and a strong and long-lasting stream of mist that distributes the oil effectively. Ideally, you want a diffuser for each room in the house.

There are two basic kinds of diffusers. An ultrasonic diffuser uses water and delivers a subtler scent. A nebulizer blows compressed air through the oil without the need for water, producing a stronger scent. It also usually has a larger capacity, meaning it can handle more rooms or a larger area. Not surprisingly, it also comes with a higher price tag. A typical cycle runs for a couple of hours before you need to reset it. Nebulizers do make a buzzing sound, but good ones allow you to turn down the mist stream, along with the sound.

All diffusers need to be cleaned after several uses. Simply wipe off any oil residue with a dry cloth or paper towel. Easy peasy!

Here are some quick and easy ways to start inhaling essential oils to help lose weight and promote abundant health.

- *Cup it.* Put a drop of citrus oil in your hand, rub your hands together, and breathe into your hands, a technique called "cupping." Citrus oils are a key ingredient in the Essential Oils Diet because they literally help your body burn fat. We'll explain how to use them in detail in chapter 6.
- *Make an impromptu steamer.* Place a couple drops of peppermint oil in a bowl of boiling water, bend over it, "tent" a towel over your head, and inhale. This will help you breathe more deeply, calm anxiety, and soothe away the pressures of life that so often trigger "stress-eating" and weight gain. Not to mention the fact that peppermint acts as an appetite suppressant!
- *Spritz it.* Fill a glass spray bottle and spritz your clothes, pillow, or the air as you would an aerosol air freshener. For every ounce of water, add ten drops of lavender essential oil, ten drops of an organic grain alcohol, and ten drops of witch hazel. This will help give your body more restorative sleep and support a proper circadian rhythm, which promotes a healthy weight.
- *On-the-go support.* Add twenty drops of any citrus oil to an aromatherapy inhaler and breathe it in whenever you feel hungry or before or during meals to manage your appetite. Keep the oil in your purse, pocket, or desk. Take four or five deep breaths when you feel hungry. You may want to close one nostril and then the other; you may want to say a little meditation or short prayer, or recite a short phrase to remind yourself of your intention to transform, to take control of your appetite. To focus, you may want to close your eyes—or not.

TOPICAL APPLICATION

Almost as safe as inhaling essential oils is applying them to your skin, if you do so properly. Topical application is the second most common way to harness the oils' healing power, and dilution is essential for both safety and efficacy.

TRY FOR YOURSELF: MAKE AN INHALER

Place ten drops of grapefruit and ten drops of lime essential oils in a glass bowl. Using a pair of tweezers, swirl an organic cotton swab in the mixture until it has slightly changed color and absorbed all the oil. Alternatively, place a cotton pad designed for aromatherapy inhalers in the glass tube of the inhaler and add the oil. Replace the clip-on cap on the glass tube. When the oil is used up, wash it out and reuse.

Both inhalers and cotton pads are readily available at many health food stores and online retailers like Amazon.com. Once created, your inhaler can last up to one year, depending on how often you open it up and use it; the more you open the lid, the more air the essential oils are exposed to, and the more quickly they will oxidize and evaporate.

The reason essential oils are called volatile organic compounds is because they begin to evaporate immediately. One or two drops go a long way, but in addition to the safety issue, diluting the oil with a carrier oil has several other advantages:

- It helps your body absorb the essential oil and prevents evaporation. Research has found that once diluted essential oils are applied on the skin, the individual chemical components can be detected in the bloodstream within five minutes.[25] Less really is more in this case.
- It is cost-effective. Remember, essential oils are volatile organic compounds, meaning that they easily evaporate. Diluting prevents wasteful evaporation, which happens in excess if you apply essential oils directly on your skin "neat," meaning undiluted. No joke, you're pouring your money away if you're using essential oils neat.
- It is sustainable. Manufacturing essential oils requires enormous quantities of plant material. If you use less, more people can enjoy the enormous benefits of these oils.

Depending on what you're trying to accomplish, it is generally advised that you dilute as follows:

- 0.5 to 1 percent: For children, the face, and sensitive skin such as genitals and underarms
- 2 percent: Standard adult dilution for most DIY applications
- 3 to 5 percent: For chronic conditions like aches and pains
- 5 to 10 percent: For acute conditions like burns and cuts and for specifically treating a disease for up to one week at a time
- 10 percent plus: To be used with great care and only for a very short period of time
- 25 percent plus: To be used only under the supervision of a trained health-care provider

Here's a quick guide to knowing how many drops of essential oil (EO) to add to achieve these percentages of dilution:

	% DILUTION	EO DROPS PER OUNCE	EO DROPS PER TABLESPOON
Infants and children	0.5%	3	1.5
	1.0%	6	3
Adults	2.0%	12	6
	3.0%	18	9
	5.0%	30	15
	10.0%	60	30

Note: There are 2 tablespoons in 1 ounce. Mix the essential oil with the carrier, then apply as indicated by the recipe or remedy for that particular ailment. You've now successfully diluted your essential oil and can enjoy the added benefit of a nourishing carrier oil.

Try for Yourself: Next time you get out of the shower, moisturize your body with a fat-burning orange body oil by mixing 2 drops of orange essential oil with 1 teaspoon of coconut oil.

Safety Note: Chemicals in some essential oils, particularly those in the citrus family, can make your skin more photosensitive; they are known as photosensitizers. (See a list of these oils below.) For example, when oils that contain bergapten are applied to the skin and then exposed to the sun, the effect of ultraviolet (UV) rays can be amplified, making the skin more susceptible to sunburn and age spots. You may simply choose not to use any oils with a lot of bergapten in them on your skin. However, you can also just avoid going out in the sun after use, or apply them only in the evening. Or use steam-distilled citrus oils, which have a lower concentration of bergapten.

PHOTOSENSITIZERS	
ESSENTIAL OIL	*LATIN NAME*
Angelica root	*Angelica archangelica*
Bergamot	*Citrus bergamia*
Bitter orange, expressed	*Citrus aurantium*
Cumin	*Cuminum cyminum*
Grapefruit	*Citrus paradisi*
Lemon, expressed	*Citrus limon*
Lime, expressed	*Citrus aurantifolia*
Rue	*Ruta graveolens*

NONPHOTOTOXIC CITRUS OILS	
ESSENTIAL OIL	*LATIN NAME*
Bergamot: Bergaptenless*	*Citrus bergamia*
Lemon, distilled	*Citrus limon*
Lime, distilled	*Citrus aurantifolia*
Mandarin	*Citrus reticulata*
Sweet or wild orange	*Citrus sinensis*
Tangelo	*Citrus tangelo*
Tangerine, expressed	*Citrus reticulata*
Yuzu oil	*Citrus junos*

* A specially formulated bergamot essential oil with the bergapten removed so it is safe to use in the sun. From Tisserand and Young's *Essential Oil Safety.*[26]

Safety Tip: Be extremely careful when using citrus oils during the summer and particularly with children, but don't feel you can't use them. Many aromatherapists agree that as long as citrus oils are heavily diluted, the risk of photosensitivity is minimal.

INGESTION

As long as they are pure and unadulterated, most essential oils that you'll find on the market are safe to consume. Some aromatherapists say that oils should never be consumed, and most will add that you should do so only under the care of a professional. But understand this: without knowing it, most people consume essential oils on a daily basis. What do you think flavors processed foods? Practically anything that is naturally or artificially flavored contains essential oils as ingredients, although food manufacturers just use microdoses, which will not afford a therapeutic benefit.

Not all essential oils are suitable for consumption, but those useful for weight control are. Not surprisingly, citrus, peppermint, herbs, and spice oils, all of which have culinary uses, are very safe for internal use. Also critical is the quantity of oil. A little peppermint oil in some fair-trade organic coffee (along with a few drops of liquid stevia and some coconut milk) is wonderfully refreshing, whereas too much peppermint can produce acid reflux.

And there are other caveats:

1. Never put undiluted essential oils in your mouth, which could burn the mucous membranes. Instead, place two or three drops in a vegan gelatin capsule diluted with an edible carrier oil such as olive, coconut, or avocado oil.
2. Don't overdo it. Use no more than three or four drops per application, and be sure to wait at least four hours before taking another dose.
3. Listen to your body.
4. Discontinue use *immediately* if you experience any adverse reactions such as nausea, acid reflux, or a headache.

Many of the food recipes that we feature in Part 3 are built around "culinary doses" of essential oils. Primarily formulated to enhance the flavor of your foods in quantities that are safe for the entire family, this strategy makes it easy for you to incorporate the natural fat-burning, healing benefits without more effort.

Try for Yourself: Put a drop of grapefruit oil and one dropperful of vanilla-flavored liquid stevia extract into a 32-ounce glass bottle and fill it with sparkling water. The carbonation will help you feel satiated, and the bioactive compounds that make up the grapefruit oil will help prompt fat-burning!

Safety Tip: If you are using any prescription medications, taking essential oils internally could put you at risk of a drug interaction. Consult your health-care provider before ingesting essential oils if you're taking pharmaceutical or over-the-counter drugs.

For more aromatherapy use guides and safety tips, and to dive deeper into how to use essential oils for everything from preventing and treating disease to making your own body-care and home-cleaning products, we recommend picking up Dr. Z's first book, *The Healing Power of Essential Oils*. It is available everywhere books are sold and at HealingPowerOfEssentialOils.com.

Mama Z here. I've been using essential oils for more than twenty-five years. My mother is a culinary herbal expert, and her best friend was a Chippewa Indian who specialized in Ojibwa and holistic medicine and used essential oils. When I was in the seventh grade, she gave me my first kit of essential oils and a book about aromatherapy. My mother wasn't interested in essential oils, but I sure was. At an early age I was also in charge of her business, so when she spoke at herbal conventions, I had the opportunity to meet a lot of people who used herbal medicines. It was a blessing to learn from holistic speakers from all over the world.

Dr. Z here. Mama Z is a total DIY guru. After we got married, she gave our home a complete essential oils makeover. We are now the parents of four young children, so we know all about "busy." But trust us, we can quickly show how you can use essential oils to enhance your health—and that definitely includes achieving a healthy weight.

You'll learn how to incorporate essential oils into super-quick recipes for delicious dishes, as well as for body-care products. Mama Z has created a great lotion with several essential oils that helps eliminate belly fat. She has also crafted homemade household cleansers that use essential oils, so you can ditch the toxin-filled products from the supermarket.

Did you know that using such products, which are full of estrogenic compounds, can actually impact your weight? You'll learn why in chapter 8.

GET READY: THE BARE ESSENTIALS

To help you get ready for your introduction to the Essential Oils Diet, you'll need to stock up on the basics. First, you'll want to get the four essential oils that support weight loss by curbing appetite and/or stimulating fat-burning, namely grapefruit, lime, peppermint, and cinnamon. We'll explain how to find an essential oils brand that works for you in chapter 6. Be sure to get all four essential oils, which are all relatively inexpensive and can be used in meals as well as in diffusers, inhalers, sprays, and topically.

Additionally, Amazon and other online retailers are excellent sources for all your aromatherapy supplies, but if you have a good organic market or health food store nearby, you may be able to find them locally.

Carrier Oils

Most essential oils are so concentrated that you should not ingest them undiluted or apply them directly to your body. Instead, mix a small amount with a carrier oil such as extra-virgin olive oil or coconut oil.

Inhalers and Other Containers

Once you start blending essential oils, you'll need containers in which to store them. There are several options:

- Aromatherapy inhaler tubes—they look like plastic lip balm containers—are great for taking a quick whiff of a single essential oil or a blend.
- For massage blends, get dark-tinted glass bottles with screw-on tops in various sizes.
- Glass bottles with spray tops in several sizes work well for air fresheners, hand sanitizers, and other spritzes. Get 1-, 8-, and 16-ounce bottles, for sure.
- For convenient, on-the-go access to your favorite healing remedies and essential oils for weight-loss recipes, 10-milliliter roller bottles work well.
- Use larger storage containers, preferably glass, but otherwise of polyethylene terephthalate (PET) plastic, which is not known to be a hormone disruptor. Look for the numeral 1 on the base to be sure.
- An ultrasonic "steam" diffuser disperses minute doses of essential oils and water into the air that find their way into your respiratory system.

CHAPTER 3

IT'S NOT YOUR FAULT: YOU'VE BEEN MISINFORMED

"Then you will know the truth, and the truth will set you free."
—JOHN 8:32

In spite of spending more money on health care than ever before, we are in the midst of a worldwide epidemic of overweight and increasing obesity, along with epidemics of cancer, metabolic syndrome—a cluster of conditions including excess abdominal fat, abnormal cholesterol levels, high blood sugar, and increased blood pressure—heart disease, type 2 diabetes, and other conditions associated with excess pounds. If you fall in this group, know that you are not alone. But with all the scientific advances of the last century, why as a society are we so sick and so heavy?

The simple answer is we have been focused on all the wrong things, ignoring the *quality* of food and fixating on the *quantity*. In other words, we've been trained to focus on non-bioactive compounds and, in our obsession with counting calories, carbs, ounces, and grams of gluten, fat, and even vitamins and minerals, we are missing the forest for the trees. As a result, falsehoods have obscured the facts. This willful ignorance of food quality by the powers that be actually encourages overeating in a fruitless effort to feel truly satisfied.

Information Overload

If you are confused about which foods belong in a healthy diet, you're not alone. A deluge of downright fake information fills books, magazine articles, and especially the Internet. Let's clear away the cobwebs obscuring the truth about the intersection of food and human metabolism. We'll start by dispelling some of the common misconceptions about what constitutes healthy food by scrutinizing eight so-called health foods, which are actually among the unhealthiest foods on the face of the earth.

The Awful Eight So-Called Health Foods

1. PUBLIC ENEMY #1: SOY PROTEIN

Unfermented soy, found in soy milk, edamame, protein powder, and countless other food products, is definitely not the same as nutritious fermented soy foods full of bioactive compounds. Think miso, natto, tempeh, and tamari. What's the difference?

- Raw soybeans are considered antinutrients for several reasons, mainly because they are trypsin-inhibitors and contain phytic acid. Trypsin is an enzyme that helps break down protein, thus contributing to vitamin B_{12} deficiency. Phytic acid prevents the absorption of minerals, especially calcium, iron, and zinc.[1]
- Fermenting soy, however, reduces these antinutrients and helps make the nutritious components of soybeans more bioavailable.[2]
- Nearly 100 percent of soy produced in the United States contains genetically modified organisms (GMOs) and has been doused with glyphosate (Roundup) to repel insects "naturally."

- The dangers of GMOs cannot be discredited, having been associated with liver and kidney problems among other health concerns.[3]
- Long-term use of soy protein powder has been connected to bladder, breast, and endometrial cancer, as well as kidney disease, underactive thyroid, asthma, cystic fibrosis, and hay fever,[4] for starters.

2. DEATH FOOD, NOT HEALTH FOOD: CONVENTIONAL MEAT

Regardless of whether it is a lean or a fatty cut, nonorganic, non-pastured beef and other meats are an absolute no-no healthwise. Remember, you are what you eat, as well as what you ate. All those hormones, pesticides, drugs, and GMOs enter your gastrointestinal (GI) tract and are stored in your fat cells.

- The natural diet of cows is grass and other plants, but conventional dairy farmers force-feed their herds GMO grains and soy full of pesticides, plus an added hit of hormones to fatten them up and an antibiotic chaser.[5]
- Unable to easily digest this unnatural diet, cows are dosed with antacids to address acid reflux and gassiness.

Additionally, the way factory farms treat animals is unequivocally antithetical to how we are directed to treat animals in the Bible: "The righteous care for the needs of their animals, but the kindest acts of the wicked are cruel" (*Proverbs 12:10*); "Six days you are to do your work, but on the seventh day you shall cease from labor so that your ox and your donkey may rest" (*Exodus 23:12*). Pick up John Robbins's seminal work *The Food Revolution* to get a clear insight into how animals are treated in factory farms. It's deplorable, and we shouldn't support that abusive behavior by buying meat products produced at the hands of torturers.

To ensure you are buying safe meat, check that the label says "grass-fed." To go one better, purchase meat and poultry from a reliable local source, such as a CSA (community supported agriculture) membership or a local farm. Buying in bulk also brings down the price of pastured beef or lamb, and sharing a side of beef with one or more friends or neighbors can cut the cost as well.

3. FARMED FISH IS FULL OF POISONS

Just like farmed meat, no way is farmed fish a "health food." Tilapia is the worst, but even farmed salmon is poison because of the GMO fish meal on which it is raised. What else is in farmed fish?

- According to an independent laboratory test commissioned by the Environmental Working Group (EWG), "seven of ten farmed salmon purchased at grocery stores in Washington, D.C., San Francisco, and Portland, Oregon, were found to be contaminated with polychlorinated biphenyls (PCBs) at levels that raise health concerns."[6] PCBs are formed by electrical transformers in the process of making plastics and certain oils.
- Farmed salmon is sixteen times more likely to contain PCBs than wild-caught varieties, four times more than beef, and at least three times more than other seafood.[7]
- Known neurotoxins and carcinogens, including dieldrin and toxaphene (both banned pesticides), dioxins, and industrial by-products from waste-treatment plants are also found in farmed fish products such as fish oil supplements.[8, 9]

4. STORE-BOUGHT FRUIT JUICE: SUGAR BY ANY OTHER NAME

Unlike eating whole fruit, which contains both soluble and insoluble fiber, drinking store-bought fruit juice every day is the antithesis of a health habit, especially if the juice comes from concentrate! In fact, regularly consuming store-bought OJ or other fruit juice actually puts you at greater risk for developing certain health problems and gaining weight. How so?

- Most conventional juices have been pasteurized to kill bacteria, destroying vitamins and minerals and leaving just flavored fructose.
- Drinking lots of juice can spike your blood glucose (sugar), followed by a blood glucose "crash," which can prompt the need for another sweet "hit," setting you up for a glucose/insulin cycle that could lead to diabetes. When your body cannot process all this extra sugar, it converts it to fat.
- Ongoing sugar spikes and crashes (hyperglycemia) can impact your insulin levels, setting the stage for developing metabolic disorders.
- Soluble and insoluble fiber in whole fruit aids digestion, makes you feel "full," and feeds the probiotics in your gut. Not so with juice.

THE "LIGHT" SIDE OF JUICE

To simply say that "juice is bad for you" and leave it at that would be a disservice because of the many beneficial nutritive qualities in freshly squeezed fruit and vegetable juices. Fresh juice contains a copious amount of vitamins, minerals, and bioactive compounds such as antioxidants that are highly bioavailable. Bottom line: If you want to load up on nutrition, consume freshly squeezed fruit or vegetable juice, especially if you're battling a cold, flu, or even cancer or another life-threatening disease.

Numerous accounts abound of cancer patients achieving favorable results while on the Gerson Therapy, which requires them to drink more than a dozen glasses of fruit and vegetable juice a day.[10] But does this mean that we all should drink a ton of juice to prevent cancer? No, not quite. Fresh fruit and vegetable juice can be a tasty treat and a great source of nutrition but need to be balanced with eating whole foods and consumed in moderation.

5. THE "VEGETABLE" OIL HOAX
AND MARGARINE MYTH

So-called vegetable oils—we can thank some clever marketer for this misleading name—are actually extracted from seeds, meaning soybeans, rapeseed (canola), corn, sunflower, cotton and safflower seeds, and peanuts. And don't let that name fool you into thinking they are healthy foods. Not in any sense of the word. Canola, corn, cotton, and soybeans are widely genetically modified.[11] Unless they are organic, all four plants have been doused with pesticides.

- They also contain extremely high levels of polyunsaturated fats. These oxidize easily, causing inflammation and cell mutations that can impact numerous health issues, including cancer, heart disease, endometriosis, and polycystic ovary syndrome.[12]
- Unlike olives or coconut, seeds cannot be cold-pressed to render oil efficiently. Instead, toxic oils such as canola and soy are heated to a high temperature, treated with a hexane solvent to extract the oil (though traces remain in the oil even after considerable refining), and finally deodorized to remove omega-3 fatty acids, which are the healthy fats we need to live, but which tend to go rancid at high temperatures.[13,14,15] Yuck!
- Because of how they are treated, vegetable oils are notoriously rich in heart-damaging trans fats. University of Florida at Gainesville researchers found trans-fat levels as high as 4.6 percent in soybean and canola oils purchased in the United States.[16] How oils subjected to such a process can be called "heart healthy" is beyond comprehension. In addition to the big problems of our time—cancer, heart disease,[17] and obesity[18,19]—these industrial oils have been linked to reproductive problems, low birth weight, hormonal issues,[20] mental decline,[21] and liver problems.[22,23]

We can't believe that we're still talking about margarine as a healthier choice than butter. Surely the "margarine myth" was laid to rest more than a decade ago. Margarine is NOT healthy. Period. So, why does the Mayo Clinic,[24] for one, argue that it is better than butter? Its logic follows:

- Margarine is made from so-called vegetable oils and therefore contains no cholesterol.
- Margarine is also higher in "good" fats—polyunsaturated and monounsaturated fats—than butter. These fats help reduce low-density lipoprotein (LDL), or "bad," cholesterol, when substituted for the saturated fat found in butter, which contains cholesterol and high levels of saturated fat.

Unfortunately, this argument simplifies and obfuscates the reality.

- Margarine is sourced from trans fats, also called trans-unsaturated fatty acids, a type of unsaturated fat that occurs in small amounts in plant-based foods but became widely available in the food supply when margarine, fried foods, and packaged baked goods were introduced in the mid-twentieth century. Trans fats have a reputation for causing cardiovascular disease and are linked to increases in type 2 diabetes and other severe health problems.[25]
- A loophole allows manufacturers to claim that a product has "0 grams of *trans* fats" if it actually contains less than 0.5 gram per serving.
- Trans fats are found not just in margarine but also in many processed foods, so they can sneak into your system even if you avoid margarine.
- To spot trans fats in processed foods, check the ingredient facts panel for "partially hydrogenated oils."

Butter, on the other hand, has not been associated with cardiovascular disease or stroke if consumed in moderation. Four studies including eleven country-specific cohorts and comprising 201,628 participants reported on butter consumption and the onset of type 2 diabetes. The finding showed that daily butter consumption of $\frac{1}{2}$ ounce (or 1 table-spoon) was associated with a lower incidence of type 2 diabetes.[26]

6. ARTIFICIAL SWEETENERS ARE UP TO NO GOOD

Another bogus health food, artificial sweeteners such as saccharine, su-cralose, and aspartame spell trouble. Who would even think the term *artificial* could coexist with the word *healthy*? Doctors still recommend them because they are allegedly "safer" for diabetics than sugar,[27] but they are anything but safe.

- Emerging research has shown that artificial sweeteners cause a disturbance in gut flora and can actually cause diabetes![28]
- Artificial sweeteners have also been linked to a laundry list of health problems, including allergies, seizures, headaches, hypertension, brain tumors, breast and bladder cancer, lymphomas and leukemia, and phenylketonuria.[29]
- Regularly eating or drinking sugar substitutes causes people to crave sweeter foods more often, thus (ironically) linking artificial sweeteners to weight gain and obesity![30]

7. PASS ON MICROWAVE POPCORN

It is touted as a healthy and convenient snack, but we cannot warn you strongly enough against consuming microwave popcorn. It is packed with carcinogens, a high price to pay for convenience. Even if you are eating a certified organic brand without GMOs, stop ASAP!

- Microwavable bags are coated with polytetrafluoroethylene (PFOA), a chemical linked to cancer.[31] Teflon is a brand name for PFOA.
- The fake butter flavoring contains a compound called diacetyl, which can cause a serious lung disease that is a form of obstructive bronchitis, as well as inflaming the nose, larynx, trachea, and bronchi when inhaled in large quantities.[32]

*To make your own popcorn, start with organic popcorn. Melt
3 tablespoons of organic coconut oil or organic butter in a heavy
stainless-steel pan. Place 2 popcorn kernels in the pan. When
one pops, pour in $1/3$ cup of popcorn and cover the pan. Shake it
occasionally to let out the steam and avoid burning the popcorn.
When the popping stops, put the popcorn in a bowl and add organic
nutritional yeast, garlic powder, cayenne pepper, or your favorite
topping.*

8. FORGET CONVENTIONAL DAIRY MILK

Long regarded as a "health food," most milk definitely does not "do
a body good." Once more, the dangers of milk lurk in the production process and cows' nutrition. Most dairy cows are fed GMO feed,
not grass and hay. Artificial hormones (rBGH) are still used to increase
milk production, although according to a 2007 Department of Agriculture study, only 17 percent of cows were injected with that hormone.[33] Use of this hormone in cows is banned throughout Europe
and in many other countries.[34]

- Toxins in dairy products have been linked to obesity,[35] early
  onset of puberty,[36] and breast and prostate cancers.[37,38]
- Pasteurizing raw milk destroys its nutritional content,
  including the enzyme lactase, which most people need to
  digest the milk protein lactose. The National Institute of
  Health reports that "approximately 65 percent of the human
  population has a reduced ability to digest lactose after
  infancy."[39]

Bottom line: Raw milk is healthier. Look for unpasteurized cheese
or yogurt products in your local health food store.

The Gluten Misconceptions

"But as for you, take wheat, barley, beans, lentils, millet and spelt, put them in one vessel and make them into bread for yourself; you shall eat it according to the number of the days that you lie on your side, three hundred and ninety days" *(Ezekiel 4:9)*. Any discussion about health myths would be incomplete without at least mentioning one of the most controversial of them all: gluten.

As biblical health educators, one question that we hear regularly is "How could gluten-containing grains such as wheat be bad for us when the Bible repeatedly refers to their consumption?" Good question. Grains have gotten a bad rap in recent years, thanks to the current obsession with the deleterious effects of the plant protein gluten.

First off, true intolerance to gluten is a very serious condition found in the small segment of the population that suffers from celiac disease, also known as celiac sprue. Such people simply cannot process gluten, which damages their intestinal lining. However, less than 1 percent of the American population has celiac disease, gluten ataxia, or even a wheat allergy.[40]

It is, therefore, surprising to learn that a recent National Public Radio (NPR) survey revealed that a whopping "29 percent of the adult population says, 'I'd like to cut back or avoid gluten completely.'"[41]

Keep in mind that gluten is big business. More than $15.5 billion of gluten-free foods were sold in 2016, which makes the truth pretty difficult to find because there is research to support both pro- and anti-gluten lifestyles.[42] Gluten awareness has been so successful that even people without gluten sensitivity avoid gluten as a preventative measure.

One thing that we can say with certainty is that a vast majority of the gluten-free products on the market sold today are absolute rubbish, filled with preservatives, sugar, and even conventional dairy. Many also contain GMO soy or grains that have been treated with glyphosate and/or contain "vegetable" oils. You can put "gluten-free" on a bottle of water and it'll sell like gluten-free hotcakes. (Pun intended, of course!) On the other hand, we have found certain gluten-free products that meet our criteria for healthy food. You'll find a number of these in our list of pantry staples and as recipe ingredients in Part 3.

GLUTEN IS STILL ON TRIAL

The jury is still out on gluten. A 2018 literature review published in the journal *Gastroenterology & Hepatology* portrays one of the more balanced evaluations of the potential risks and benefits of a gluten-free diet (GFD).[43] A summary of their findings follows.

POTENTIAL BENEFITS AND HARMS OF A GFD IN NON-CELIAC DISEASE PATIENTS

Conditions with Potential Benefits from a GFD	Potential Harms of a GFD
Gluten-sensitive irritable bowel syndrome	Deficiencies of micronutrients and fiber
Nonceliac gluten sensitivity	Increases in fat content of foods
Schizophrenia or other mental health conditions	Hyperlipidemia
Atopy	Hyperglycemia
Fibromyalgia	Coronary artery disease
Endometriosis	Social impairment or restrictions
Obesity	
Athletic performance	

Humans have existed on wheat and other gluten-containing grains since the beginning of recorded history. Why are these grains vilified today? Is gluten bad for everyone? Most people assume that the issue has been put to bed. But is it true? Is gluten itself the problem? Or is this yet another misstep in nutrition history?

Only time will tell, but something tells us that there's more to the story than that which presently meets the eye.

Contrary to popular belief, wheat and other gluten-containing products may not be bad in and of themselves. There is actually a growing body of evidence that suggests gluten isn't unhealthy at all and has shouldered the blame for so-called gluten reactions that are actually a response to the toxins used in conventional farming. Wheat farmers drench their fields with the weed killer glyphosate (Roundup) before the harvest, which causes the wheat to go to seed before it dies, unnaturally boosting the crop. The treatment also allows the wheat field to ripen all at once, requiring only one pass with the thresher, and simultaneously kills the competing rye grass, eliminating a major weed problem. Glyphosate is also used on soybeans. Soy, like wheat, is a ubiquitous ingredient in processed foods.

According to Dr. Stephanie Seneff, a senior research scientist at the Massachusetts Institute of Technology, this dangerous farming practice has been linked to a wide variety of diseases, and it is also the real reason so many people are gluten intolerant and have celiac disease. Dr. Seneff and her colleagues have proven beyond a shadow of a doubt that glyphosate—not gluten or GMO wheat—which has been banned in most European countries since 2015,[44] annihilates gut flora and leads to the chronic inflammation typical of gluten-related autoimmune diseases and other ailments.[45,46]

Additionally, it's important to note that today's wheat and gluten-bearing grains aren't the same crops that our ancestors ate. For thousands of years, we cultivated grains, stored them, milled them, and consumed them as a primary source of food. Grains were soaked, sprouted, and fermented, and bread was baked using slow-rise yeast, all of which increases the grain's nutritional content and bioavailability.[47,48] When farming technology was invented during the industrial era, things changed, and quantity was given precedence over quality.[49]

In addition to countless unnatural growing techniques, farmers started to overharvest the land, not letting it rest as the Bible mandates, and soil nutrition (and subsequent crops) started to decline. Grains were no longer fermented or sprouted because it took too much time, and wheat was hybridized to contain unnatural amounts of gluten for making soft, chewy, and fluffy baked goods. When bleached white flour came into vogue, the cumulative changes created a perfect storm that made most grains grown in the United States unfit for human consumption.

FAKE FOOD VS. REAL SALT

Table salt is produced from sea salt, but most harvesting methods strip away all of salt's naturally occurring minerals and replace them with additives, including aluminum. This takes salt from a "real" food to a fake food in no time, while also destroying the naturally occurring iodine and replacing it with potentially toxic levels of potassium iodide.

Also added is dextrose, which turns the salt purple. But no one wants to eat purple salt, so next a bleaching agent is used to restore the white color. Instead of this chemistry experiment, try the actual product. We recommend you start using pink Himalayan or Celtic sea salt ASAP.

Grains grown in other countries, however, have not been tampered with in the way that they have been in the States. Through a phenomenon known as the "Italian paradox," gluten-intolerant American travelers discover that they can freely eat gluten products with no side effects in many other countries.

Bottom line: Even if gluten isn't bad for us, Americans should stay away from most conventionally grown grains because of the dangers inherent in conventional farming techniques. And, just to be on the safe side, the Essential Oils Diet recommends avoiding gluten-bearing grains, particularly because of the association between gluten and potential weight gain.

It may seem like an overwhelming task to omit such foods because gluten is everywhere. Unquestionably, it requires a learning curve at first, but after a while living gluten-free is quite easy, as you'll learn in chapter 7.

WHAT MAKES A *REAL* HEALTH FOOD?

Put any food to the test by asking these questions:
- Does it promote good health, meaning its nutritional components and bioactive compounds have not been destroyed by pasteurization and other industrial processes?
- Is it as close to its natural (unprocessed) state as possible?
- Has it been raised organically without toxins, hormones, and GMOs?
- Has it avoided exposure to toxins and pollutants (due to pollution or environmental destruction)?
- Did the animal that winds up on the dinner table consume its natural diet?
- Is it locally grown or raised?

Eating most of such foods, which are inherently natural, with a few exceptions cited in this chapter, helps you achieve your ideal weight.

Misinformation About Exercise

Now let's dispel some common myths about exercise. First, exercise, as in going to the gym, jogging, or practicing hot yoga, is a great way to reduce body fat and build muscle, improving your body composition and raising your metabolism. Exercise also enhances endurance, improves respiration rates, and elevates mood. Still, exercise is not particularly effective at peeling off pounds.

Why? Because muscle tissue weighs more than an equivalent amount of fat, so muscle gain offsets fat loss. As you become more active, your metabolism assumes this is the new norm and resets your internal clock. Plus, physical activity expends energy but may also make you hungrier, neutralizing the effects of calorie burn. To see the needle on the scale move significantly, exercise alone is not enough. You will likely also have to change your eating habits.

The real value of being a body in motion is improved mood[50] and enhanced health. Lack of exercise is a major cause of heart disease and diabetes,[51] but regular cardio can improve body composition,[52] reducing such risks.[53,54] Physical fitness also reduces the likelihood of developing cancer.[55,56,57] Another major benefit: Exercise builds bone strength, reducing the risk of osteoporosis and fractures.[58]

What Counts?

Just as we do with food, we tend to quantify exercise rather than think of it qualitatively. No doubt that's why so many people regard exercise as a chore—but what could be more enjoyable than moving your body as it was designed to move, feeling your strength, and seeing your endurance building week by week? If you're focused only on doing so many push-ups or running X number of miles, or burning so many calories in a session, it can become just another item on your to-do list. And your initial enthusiasm may wane.

To watch Mama Z discuss her exercise regimen and show you how to properly perform the exercises that we recommend in the Essential Oils Diet, visit EssentialOilsDiet.com.

Your Fitbit or similar device can motivate you to walk another few thousand steps a day, but does it take into consideration whether you're jogging on a treadmill in a noisy gym or on a quiet nature trail, whether you're plugged into earphones or talking with a good buddy? Of course not. And don't forget that horsing around with your kids counts—on more levels than one. Bottom line: For regular exercise to become a habit, one that transforms your body and your mind-set, it has to be enjoyable.

The Myth of a Longer Life Span

Think of sitting as the new smoking.[59] There's no question that our industrialized lifestyle is killing us, causing weight gain, diabetes, multiple other health problems, and decreased life expectancy. We are *not* actually living longer. The real reason the stats on average life span seem to have improved is that fewer children die in infancy, raising the mean age.[60]

Nor are we necessarily living better. Consider the quality of life that all too often characterizes old age. Consuming lots of prescription drugs, enduring pain and reduced mobility, and perhaps even suffering from Alzheimer's and other forms of dementia are no way to spend your "golden years."

Lessons from the Blue Zones

Dan Buettner, author of *The Blue Zones* and companion titles, has studied cultures around the globe with the longest life expectancy, specifically Sardinia, Okinawa in Japan, the Nicoya peninsula of Costa Rica, the Greek island of Ikaria, and Loma Linda, a small California city that is home to many Seventh-Day Adventists. These far-flung populations do not engage in so-called exercise. Nor do they need to: their way of life involves regular and constant motion. They also tend to be slim, in large part because their diets are primarily plant-based.

The five Blue Zone populations do not all eat the same foods, but they do share certain dietary patterns. They are generally locavores, eating the food raised nearby, and little or no animal protein. Most Loma Linda Seventh-Day Adventists are vegetarians—some are vegans—and some occasionally eat fish and/or poultry. Other populations rely primarily on fish for their protein needs. Sardinians eat lots of anchovies and olive oil, both of which are full of healthful omega-3 fats, often flavored with rosemary. As islanders, Okinawans and Ikarians also rely on fish. Legumes are staples in all five Blue Zones, as are vegetables, fruits, and a variety of ancient grains such as oatmeal, quinoa, millet, brown rice, spelt, amaranth, sorghum, and teff. Processed sugar and processed foods are not on any menu.

In addition, the individuals in Blue Zones generally share other life-enhancing and life-extending patterns:

- They have a purpose, a reason to get up in the morning.
- They have ways to decompress, to relax, whether via prayer, activity, or socializing.
- They are part of a tribe of like-minded people.
- Family comes first.
- They are engaged in their community.
- They have a belief in some higher power.

Seventh-Day Adventists are particularly interesting as they live in a city in the most populous state in the country, not on a self-contained island or peninsula where life hasn't changed much for generations. As the longest-lived Americans, they set the bar for how to live in the modern world without buying into a lifestyle that equates with compromised health and a reduced life span. This has made the Adventists an ideal subject of longitudinal research. One study looked at the impact on life span of the three protein consumption patterns. It comes as no surprise that the vegan Adventists tend to live the longest, followed by the vegetarians, and finally those who occasionally consume animal protein.[61]

Marketing and Misinformation

In summary, the agricultural, chemical, and pharmaceutical industries have messed with your health—and the health of millions of others—as well as your mind by foisting unhealthy products on the public. The movers and shakers in these industries may have initially been well intentioned as they developed new processes, new food additives, new drugs, new insecticides, and on and on. Most conventionally trained doctors signed on and turned a blind eye, or simply didn't realize the implications of such dramatic changes and their potential to impact the health of their patients.

Nonetheless, the law of unintended consequences has produced a massive problem.

In effect, we humans are the guinea pigs in a gigantic scientific experiment. What does a lifetime of consuming and being exposed to new substances do to us (to say nothing of the animals that provide much of what we consume)? The jury is still out, and the experiment is ongoing as chemists churn out more and more substances.

We do know that most food, and particularly processed food, is full of unnatural and often toxic additives, stabilizers, and other ingredients. We intuitively understand that most fast food contains dubious ingredients. Otherwise, how could it be so cheap?

You also may not be quite so aware of the barrage of toxins in household cleaners, synthetic carpets and upholstery, hand wipes, and countless other products. Many of these chemicals contain xenohormones that can interact with your hormones and exacerbate your struggle with weight. Fortunately, once you know where these toxins are hiding (often in plain sight), you can eliminate many of them. The health properties of essential oils also help to negate or minimize the effects of environmental toxins we cannot avoid. We recommend picking up our book *The Healing Power of Essential Oils* to get all of the do-it-yourself recipes and home remedies that you'll need to completely detox your house. When you buy a copy, be sure to go to HealingPowerofEssentialOils.com to access a series of demo videos that we have recorded to help you make these recipes!

But first, it's time to introduce you to the Essential Fast Track, the first phase of the Essential Oils Diet. Turn the page to discover the *real* health foods you should be eating.

PART 2

INTRODUCING THE TRANSFORMATIONAL ESSENTIAL OILS DIET

CHAPTER 4

WHAT YOU NEED TO KNOW BEFORE YOU START THE ESSENTIAL OILS DIET

"The greatest medicine of all is to teach people not to need it."
—HIPPOCRATES

By now you understand that this book is unlike any other book on health and diet you have ever read. To our knowledge, no other weight-loss program incorporates essential oils as a weight-loss aid via food and capsule recipes, inhalation, and topical applications, while also focusing on bioactive-rich foods. When you transform your body and its relationship to food, you throw open the door to the possibility of countless other changes, whether in your relationships, your attitude about exercise, or even your life's work.

In this chapter, we'll discuss the overall objectives of the program, and then in the following chapters, we'll get into the specifics of the two phases—the *Essential Fast Track* and the *Essential Lifestyle*—with one chapter that zeroes in on how to incorporate essential oils into the program.

When you consume bioactive compounds on a regular basis, your body achieves its natural weight. In addition to attaining a healthy weight, the objectives of the Essential Oils Diet are to soothe inflammation, reduce stress, help you overcome unhealthy food cravings, heal your gut, and put yourself in a position where you can form good habits and a healthy relationship to food that will ultimately result in transformation.

Six More Reasons You Will Succeed

The Essential Oils Diet differs from other weight-loss programs in at least six other respects.

1. IT DOESN'T OVERCOMPLICATE THINGS

It is quite simple to lose weight. You have probably done it at least once if not several times before! The trick is to *keep off* the weight by adopting new and permanent habits. We'll help you do that by prompting you to set your goals and commit to transformation. Then it's a matter of filling your fridge and pantry with healthy food, consuming it in moderation, and enlisting family and friends for support as you embark on this journey.

2. NO NEED TO COUNT ANYTHING

Forget about tracking calories or grams of carbs. Instead, eat moderate portions, stopping before you're completely full. Easier said than done, right? Well, it's not as hard as you may think.

God has designed your body with a wonderful set of checks and balances and given you hormones such as leptin to tell your brain when you should stop eating.[1,2] Here are some clues to let you know when this is happening and when you should push the plate aside, even though there may still be food on it. It's time to quit the Clean Plate Club!

- *Clue #1: Your meal starts to lose its flavor and isn't as satisfying.* The human body craves energy-rich, tasty fats and carbs when it's starving. The opposite is also true. Once your meal provides what your body needs, your cravings will quickly dissipate and you will feel sick if you overeat.
- *Clue #2: Your energy level will drop, and you'll start to get a little tired.* If you need a cup of coffee or espresso and a sugary dessert after a meal to keep you going, you have eaten too

JOURNALING IS ESSENTIAL

We can't stress enough how important it is to keep your Transformation Journal during this process of transformation. Start by listing the goals you have set for yourself—not just about your body, but for your life. Record not just what you eat each day, but also your emotions and challenges. If you fall off the wagon, this record will allow you to examine why it happened and make an immediate course correction.

For example, perhaps you didn't have a chance to get to the grocery store and fell back on your old habit of ordering take-out from a fast-food place. Instead, going forward, make sure your freezer is always filled with acceptable options to avoid a repeat, but don't beat yourself up for one misstep. Feeling guilty can lead to further problems. Remember, total health transformation is a lifelong marathon, not a quick weight-loss sprint. A few mistakes don't cancel out all of the successes that you've achieved along the way.

Once you keep track of yourself this way, you will see how you can come up with strategies that allow you to be more in control when certain situations arise. Instead of measuring your weight or your waist size, try journaling how you *feel*. Why? For two reasons.

First, your weight will vary considerably depending on the time of day—and for women where they are in their monthly cycle. Second, evaluating how your symptoms wax and wane is a better indicator of true health. Seriously, what's the point of having six-pack abs if you're constipated, depressed, and riddled with pain, right?

much. In fact, we have found that eating enough food to feel satisfied but stopping *before* your tummy feels full, as indicated by an extended, bulging belly, is a key to sustained energy that will last all day long.

- **Clue #3: You will start to feel your stomach expand.** When you feel "uncomfortable" around the middle, you've gone too far.

Take note of when you first feel your tummy push up against your belt or against the table. This will alert you next time. This is also a reason why you need to eat slowly, to give your brain a chance to receive signals from your stomach that you have eaten enough.

Soon you will recognize the difference between feeling pleasantly satisfied and feeling stuffed. The former feels comfortable; the latter does not. Likewise, all too often we confuse thirst with hunger. Stay well hydrated throughout the day by drinking plenty of healthy liquids such as tea and water.

THE DANGERS OF LEPTIN RESISTANCE

If you find it difficult to stop at that comfort point when eating, you're not alone. This can be particularly difficult for obese people because they are likely to be suffering from leptin resistance. Leptin is a hormone that sends signals to your brain that you've had enough to eat and helps monitor your weight.

When a person gorges past that comfortable sensation of "fullness," his body produces leptin in an effort to tell the brain to transmit a message to stop eating. If you repeatedly ignore these signals and continue to eat through the sensation of satiety, your body will adapt to elevated levels of leptin, ultimately making you resistant to it.[3] If you never feel satisfied, you'll always be tempted to eat more. Scary!

3. NO "GOOD" OR "BAD" FOODS

Diet programs that exclude major food groups entirely are unsustainable. Carbohydrates, fats, and protein all belong on your plate. In this book, there are no lengthy lists of good foods and bad foods to memorize or refer to frequently. With the exception of toxic ingredients—processed sugar, for example, which is lacking in any nutritive value—and foods that are industrially raised or genetically modified, almost all foods are acceptable. We do advise you to avoid a few other foods we feel are unclean or that come from polluted sources. Certain foods are best omitted until you reach your desired weight, but then they can be reintroduced.

4. WE RESPECT BIOCHEMICAL INDIVIDUALITY

The Essential Oils Diet focuses on your biochemical individuality, which means that our physiologies are as unique as our fingerprints. There is simply no one-size-fits-all approach to health and diet. You need to find what works for *your* unique biochemical makeup.

Take our family, for example. Dr. Z and our kids do exceptionally well consuming raw dairy cheese and non-GMO organic sprouted grains that contain gluten. Mama Z, on the other hand, is very sensitive to gluten and all forms of dairy. She thrives on eating more meat than Dr. Z, whose diet is 95 percent plant-based.

It's a matter of finding what works for you, and we'll walk you through how to do that.

5. EAT WHAT YOU LOVE

This is a program that capitalizes on your God-given instincts and natural, healthy desires for a wide variety of foods. We also think it's important to remember that fad diets that restrict fruits, vegetables, grains, and legumes are not only unhealthy, but they are also unbiblical: "Then God said, 'I give you every seed-bearing plant on the face of the whole earth and every tree that has fruit with seed in it. They will be yours for food'" *(Genesis 1:29).*

With these basic guidelines under your belt, there's no need for a meal plan that tells you to have a spinach salad for lunch on Monday and turkey breast for dinner on Wednesday. After all, you know whether you prefer broccoli to cauliflower—or love them both. Ditto for nectarines or strawberries. Instead of meal plans to follow slavishly, use the recipes Mama Z has provided, modify them, or substitute or modify your own recipes to conform with our short list of guidelines.

Eating the healthy foods that you prefer makes it far more likely that you'll adhere to the program—and make it a permanent way of eating. However, that's not to say that you can't experiment with some new foods. You might find you look at kale a whole new way once you have it in our Kale and Lentil Super Soup (page 236)!

6. NOT JUST FOR WEIGHT LOSS

The Essential Oils Diet is equally effective if chronic illness, an overactive thyroid, an injury, or another issue has made it difficult to gain weight or maintain a healthy weight. In this case, you can start with the Essential Lifestyle in chapter 7.

Still, it would be a good idea to skim chapter 5, as we touch on topics such as movement, fasting, and colon cleansing, which are equally applicable to the Essential Lifestyle. Likewise, if you are already at your goal weight but want to enhance your health, feel more energetic, or simply live a more natural lifestyle, you can begin with the Essential Lifestyle. In either case, be sure to complete this chapter in order to understand the fundamentals of the program.

Food vs. So-Called Food

We all love food, and much of the time it loves us back, providing energy and the nutrients vital to a long, healthy life. But food can also create digestive upset and metabolic problems. Plus, not all of the food products you see on the market are created equal. And more is definitely not better.

The foods you'll focus on in the Essential Oils Diet are rich in bioactive compounds, which as you now know are found primarily in plant foods such as vegetables, fruits, legumes, and ancient whole grains like oatmeal, quinoa, millet, brown rice, spelt, amaranth, sorghum, and teff. You'll rely on such whole foods while eliminating most processed foods, aka fake foods, starting with refined sugar. Remember, sugar is more addictive than cocaine, so we'll be tackling this challenge at length.[4]

The Food Essentials

The approach to food in the Essential Oils Diet is simple and highly adaptable to your tastes and preferences. Here are the basics:

1. First and foremost, you will be eating unprocessed or minimally processed food full of bioactive compounds.
2. Vegetables and fruit will be the major players on your plate.
    - Produce should be primarily organically grown. Locally grown produce is preferable to food transported great distances from where it was grown, often losing nutrients by the mile.
    - Consume all fruits and veggies that agree with you. For a variety of reasons such as chronic inflammation, autoimmunity, or other preexisting disorders, some people simply can't handle certain foods. Sensitive to nightshade vegetables? Then avoid eggplant, tomatoes, bell peppers, and goji berries. Can't consume gluten without getting bloated? Steer clear of it. It's really as simply as that.
    - List in your Transformation Journal all the foods to which you are sensitive. This will help remind you of what to avoid in the future and also give you a baseline against which to measure your success. If all goes as planned, none of these foods will bother you after a year or two of following the Essential Oils Diet. This is total healing, something we've not only personally experienced but have also seen happen in people that we've helped.
3. Your protein intake will come primarily from wild-caught fish, nuts, legumes, and vegetables. If you want an extra boost of protein, make a shake using Mama Z's Super Greens Powder (page 220) or Living Fuel SuperGreens. More on that in chapter 5.
    - As we see in the Bible and most other sacred texts, our ancestors occasionally ate small portions of pastured meat

and free-range poultry. (Of course, they didn't call it that in those days!)

- The excessive consumption of meat championed by the low-carb, high-fat, ketogenic, and Paleo crazes has been shown to cause disease such as nonalcoholic fatty liver disease and insulin resistance.[5] Researchers in France have been so bold as to point out that "a high-fat diet has also been shown to be a good model to simulate human metabolic syndrome!"[6] Trust us, a heavy meat diet is not sustainable for you—or the planet. Not to mention, the weight-loss benefits are oftentimes short-lived on such diets.[7,8]

4. That said, the Essential Oils Diet is perfectly adaptable for those who prefer a completely plant-based diet.

5. Moderation is key. Too much of a good thing is still "too much," right? If you gorge on healthy snacks, you'll end up gaining weight, so eat until you feel pleasantly full but not stuffed. Revisit the section on page 70 to learn how to gauge your appetite.

6. Fast regularly. In the next chapter, we'll offer you a host of options from skipping a single meal to fasting for a whole day. Pick the one that works best for you initially in terms of your schedule, weight-loss goals, and any specific health concerns. If setting the bar relatively low means you are more able to be compliant, by all means listen to that inner voice. But also keep your options open over time. As you come to see the benefit of intermittent fasting, you will likely be inclined to take it up a notch, then another notch!

DR. ATKINS'S GHOST STILL HAUNTS US

We get a lot of flak online about why we do not promote low-carb, high-fat diets. (The only other equally divisive topic in the natural health community is which essential oil company is the "best" brand.) We can't blame someone for following such a diet program, particularly if they attribute their diet to healing a chronic disease or helping them lose weight when nothing else could.

That said, there continues to be endless debate over the dangerously low-carb, high-fat dietary approach pioneered by Dr. Atkins, which lives on in one form or another as the South Beach diet, Wheat Belly diet, Paleo diet, and keto diet, among the myriad followers.

Think of low-carb, high-fat diets as akin to get-rich-quick pyramid schemes. They have been designed to *cheat the system* that God put in place when He designed our human physiology to consume a wide range of plant-based food. Natural gurus today refer to this as "biohacking." However, going low carb/high fat isn't natural in any sense of the word. Such programs are get-out-of-jail cards; in other words, they are short-lived. It's important to keep in mind that vegetables, fruits, legumes, and ancient grains have been part of our diet since the dawn of humanity.

One by one, these fad diets get debunked, but only after countless innocent, trusting consumers expend millions of dollars on books, supplements, and processed food products trying to find a solution to their unceasing weight problem. Take the Paleo diet, for example, which rests on the assumption that our Paleolithic ancestors never ate grains. This fallacy was debunked by the recent finding that an old Stone Age pestle was actually covered with oat starch residue, suggesting that ancient humans ground oats into flour and, presumably, dined on oatcakes or some other grain-based delicacy.[9]

The ketogenic diet rests on the ability to consume less than 5 percent of one's daily caloric intake in the form of carbohydrates. Engineered to help epileptic children in the 1920s, it is now heralded as the cure-all for everything from obesity to cancer.[10] But there have been no longitudinal studies conducted on humans to substantiate that going keto is safe as a permanent lifestyle change. Like all diets, keto should be seen as a "reset" (and a potentially dangerous one at that), but it is definitely not a long-term solution.

The Essential Eight

The following groups of foods and herbs form the core of the Essential Oils Diet. All are rich in bioactive compounds that promote overall health and encourage or support fat-burning by addressing factors such as inflammation, stress, insulin resistance, and hyperglycemia. All of these conditions can cause weight gain and interfere with weight loss. In each category, we've listed a few of our favorites, which are also the most thoroughly researched, but plenty of related foods are also replete with bioactives.

1. SEEDS

Seeds are embryonic plants and, as such, contain amazing life-enhancing properties.

- *Hempseed* is all the rage these days, but the Chinese have cooked with the oil and used it medicinally for more than 3,000 years.[11] The seeds are full of omega-3 and omega-6 essential fatty acids, as well as gamma-linolenic acid. An ounce of hempseed contains as much protein as an ounce of beef or lamb.[12] As a complete protein, it provides all the essential amino acids your body requires but cannot produce on its own. (One of the few other plants with this distinction is quinoa.) It is also a good source of vitamin E and a whole slew of minerals.[13,14]

  Hempseed is easier to digest than most grains, nuts, and legumes[15] and can reduce inflammation,[16] a factor in weight gain. Whole hempseeds are also a good source of both soluble and insoluble fiber.[17]
- *Cacao seeds* were treasured by the ancient Mayans, who thought that cacao was of divine origin. The Aztecs believed that consuming chocolate gave humans some of their god Quetzalcoatl's wisdom. Both ancient cultures also used

it medicinally. We now know that cacao is a powerful antioxidant and can help regulate the immune system, tamping down inflammation and protecting against oxidative stress.

Cacao can also offset hyperglycemia and insulin resistance, factors that promote obesity;[18] improve mitochondrial biogenesis (an essential cellular response to energy status); and modulate obesity-related inflammation caused by a high-fat diet.[19] Look for cacao nibs or sugar-free dark chocolate (72 percent or more cacao).

A PAIR OF HONORABLE MENTIONS

Chia seeds are also a great source of plant fiber. Daily consumption of 35 grams of chia flour over twelve weeks resulted in greater loss of weight and inches than in a placebo group that consumed an otherwise similar diet.[20] The chia group also saw a reduction in total cholesterol and an increase in high-density lipoprotein (HDL), or "good," cholesterol, factors that reduce cardiac risk.

Flaxseed is another hardworking dietary fiber, helping to manage your weight,[21] lower cholesterol and therefore reduce cardiovascular risk,[22] and improve insulin resistance, reducing the risk of developing type 2 diabetes.[23]

2. HEALTHY FATS AND OILS

- *Extra-virgin olive oil* is still the best overall source of fat on the planet, and its consumption as part of a nutritious diet promotes weight loss. In one study of women with breast cancer, an olive oil–enriched diet produced more weight loss than a lower-fat diet.[24] In the follow-up in six months, the subjects overwhelmingly chose the former.

The predominant fatty acid in olives is an extremely healthy monounsaturated fat known as oleic acid. Shown to reduce inflammation, consuming oleic acid can help with virtually every inflammatory chronic disease, including cancer,[25] autoimmunity,[26] and dementia.[27] Olive oil is also rich in antioxidants, which can have profound healing effects on the body.[28] A meta-analysis of forty-two reports including 841,211 people strongly suggests that regularly consuming olive oil reduces mortality risk, risk of a cardiovascular event, and even risk of stroke.[29]

- *Avocado oil* contains a high level of monounsaturated fat, making it a winner in the weight-loss department and providing the trifecta of lowering cholesterol, banishing hunger pangs, and spot-reducing fat around the middle. The latter is a known risk factor for the metabolic syndrome. This "olive oil of the Americas" has a high smoke point, meaning it doesn't oxidize at high temperatures.

  Although antioxidants in vegetables and fruits can combat some of the free radicals in your body, they can't reach your mitochondria, which play a key role in keeping your metabolism on track. Consuming avocado oil and other monounsaturated fats helps mitochondria survive attack from free radicals.[30] It does you little good to eat foods full of bioactive compounds if your body can't absorb them. Avocado oil and other oils high in monounsaturated fats are necessary to carry those carotenoids and other bioactive compounds into your bloodstream. In fact, research suggests that consuming 20 grams of monounsaturated fatty acid–rich oils—or four and a half teaspoons, which is roughly the average serving of oil in most vinaigrettes—during your meals is required for optimal carotenoid absorption.[31]

  So, you don't need to drown your salad or stir-fry in avocado oil to get maximum absorption of those important compounds. We'll get into other ways avocados help you lose weight on page 82.

3. FRUIT

As long as you don't experience a negative reaction due to an allergy, all fruit is safe on the Essential Oils Diet. Note, however, if you're trying to lose excess weight, you may want to eat high-sugar fruits such as apples, pears, and pineapple sparingly, at least during the Essential Fast Track. Once you reach a healthy weight that you are happy with and find your groove in the Essential Lifestyle phase, you can enjoy these fruits in larger quantities without giving much thought to putting on extra pounds.

- *Berries,* whether strawberries, blueberries, raspberries, blackberries, loganberries, or others, are packed with a host of bioactive components, including anthocyanins, a type of flavonoid, which give foods their pigments. Plus, all those tiny seeds are a great source of fiber, which you already know can depress appetite.

  A midafternoon snack of mixed berries (a serving of just under 1 cup) has been shown to reduce the amount of food consumed at dinner a few hours later.[33] Researchers now realize that such positive effects as improved brain, visual, and vascular functions, and particularly anti-diabetes and anti-obesity impacts, cannot be ascribed solely to the antioxidant properties of berries, prompting further research into bioactivity.[34]

- *Avocado.* Wait a minute. Didn't we just talk about avocados? Indeed, this poster child for healthy eating—and, yes, it is a fruit—deserves double billing. Just adding avocado to a salad lets you absorb three to five times the amount of carotenoids[35] in the other ingredients.

  Eating half a Hass avocado (the small dark kind with a rough skin) at lunchtime has been shown to produce a 40 percent decreased desire to eat for several hours afterward.[36] That daily half avocado has also been shown to help with several other positive indicators for ongoing weight management and is associated with a lower body mass index (BMI) and smaller waist, reducing the risk for metabolic syndrome by 50 percent.[37] Avocados are also good sources of fiber and provide much of your daily need for vitamin K, both of which help with weight control by regulating sugar metabolism and insulin sensitivity.

DR. Z TIP

Avocados are a must in my morning smoothie. They make it super creamy and so nutritious. A salad made from dark leafy greens, the densest source of vitamin K, and a few slices of avocado or a dollop of guacamole can eliminate the blood sugar roller coaster that could prompt you to head for the cookie jar. More good news: Eating some avocado before a workout provides an energy boost that lets you work a bit harder,[38] increasing your metabolism so you burn more calories during and after your workout.

DR. Z TIP

For all its weight-loss properties, grapefruit has a darker side. Certain pharmaceuticals, such as statins, can negatively interact with this fruit because they are metabolized by the cytochrome P4503A4 enzyme found in its juice. Grapefruit inhibits this enzyme, thus rendering certain drugs less effective. However, there is no such risk with grapefruit essential oil, because this drug interaction is primarily due to dihydroxybergamottin, which is not present in the oil.[40]

4. CRUCIFEROUS VEGETABLES

Regarded as one of the healthiest food groups we can consume, cruciferous vegetables are potent anti-inflammatories, cancer fighters, and natural detoxifiers.[41,42] Cruciferous vegetables are rich in bioactive compounds such as glucosinolates, fiber, carotenoids (beta-carotene, lutein, zeaxanthin); vitamins C, E, and K; folate; and minerals, so much so that the National Institute of Health, which sponsors the National Cancer Institute, is studying cruciferous vegetables extensively because the compounds are known to do the following:[43]

- Protect cells from DNA damage
- Inactivate carcinogens

- Produce antiviral, antibacterial, and anti-inflammatory effects
- Induce cell death (apoptosis)
- Inhibit angiogenesis (tumor blood vessel formation) and tumor cell migration (which is needed for metastasis)

- *Broccoli.* You've undoubtedly heard that the dark green, leafy cruciferous veggie called kale boasts a ton of health benefits. It was actually ranked fifteenth in a Centers for Disease Control and Prevention study of forty-seven "powerhouse" fruits and vegetables.[44] But it is only one of the family members, so let's focus on some more traditional crucifers, such as broccoli. It has been the subject of plenty of research that shows its long-term consumption can counteract nonalcoholic fatty liver disease, which is known to progress to hepatocellular carcinoma, a cancer with a high mortality rate.[45] Do steer clear of prepackaged broccoli, which may have spent days in transit and in the supermarket; after processing and commercial transport, levels of bioactive compounds plummet.[46] We expect to see the same results in most bioactive-rich foods, so try to grow your own or purchase veggies from local organic farmers.
- *Bok choy,* the most popular vegetable in China, has a milder flavor than most members of the cabbage family. All contain sulforaphane, which improves blood pressure and kidney function; it also produces that distinctive odor when cabbage is overcooked. A bioactive powerhouse, bok choy boasts lutein and other such anti-inflammatory, cancer-protective tongue-twisters such as isothiocyanates, thiocyanates, and zeaxanthin, as well as vitamins A, B, and C. Bok choy is very low in calories—not that you'll be counting them on the Essential Oils Diet—thanks to its high fiber content.

To watch Mama Z make her super-healthy and tasty cruciferous veggie coleslaw, and to get more ideas on how to incorporate cruciferous vegetables into your diet, visit EssentialOilsDiet.com.

5. NUTS

Although they are calorie dense, these petite packages of protein, unsaturated fat, and fiber are nutritional powerhouses. Eating a daily handful of nuts in lieu of less healthful foods can help prevent obesity, type 2 diabetes,[47,48] and heart disease.[49,50] Most nuts are tree nuts, but peanuts and cashews are actually the seeds of legumes.

- **Almonds.** It doesn't get much better than this: Research consistently shows that daily consumption in both small (10 grams) and large (100 grams) amounts does *not* result in weight gain[51]—and even small amounts can improve health. Snacking on almonds can improve fat metabolism and moderate the rise in blood sugar level after meals[52] and increase satiety, or the pleasant feeling of fullness. Substituting just one high-carb snack such as a muffin with a handful of almonds may be enough to head off cardio-metabolic diseases even without weight loss.[53] Adding almonds to a low-calorie weight-loss program over twenty-four weeks actually resulted in more weight loss and greater improvements in markers for metabolic syndrome.[54]
- **Walnuts** offer many of the same benefits as almonds. However, walnuts contain much higher amounts of both omega-3 and omega-6 fatty acids than almonds and most other nuts, making them particularly effective in reducing the risk of type 2 diabetes.[55] Packed with bioactive antioxidants, walnuts appear to be even more effective than almonds in reducing oxidation after a meal.[56]

6. LEGUMES

The choice food of the Blue Zones, legumes, such as beans, peas, lentils, and clovers—as well as peanuts and cashews—contain bioactive components that may reduce the risk of developing cardiovascular disease and type 2 diabetes. Legumes are packed with dietary fiber and antioxidants, a dynamic duo in addressing the post-meal hyperglycemia (high blood sugar) and hyperlipidemia (excessive lipids in the blood) that follow a typical American meal. We consume far fewer legumes than do people in developing countries, to our detriment, although soy is common in many processed foods. (Note that we do not recommend soybeans or unfermented soy products, as they are almost invariably GMO.)

- *Black beans* contain bioactive compounds known as anthocyanidins that give a fruit or vegetable its color. Anthocyanidins also inhibit various metabolic responses, thereby lowering blood sugar after a meal, which is particularly important for delaying or preventing the onset of heart disease and type 2 diabetes in individuals with metabolic syndrome.[57] Regular consumption of black beans should also help prevent the development of such health problems.

- *Lentils,* also called pulses, are a nutritious food staple for millions of people who eat a mainly or completely plant-based diet. Lentils may be green, black, red, or yellow, and all contain numerous bioactive components as well as prebiotic carbohydrates, upon which your gut bacteria survive.[58] Prebiotic carbohydrates and dietary fiber both have the potential to reduce the risks of becoming obese or developing cancer, heart disease, and diabetes.

A DYNAMIC DUO: LENTILS AND KALE

Lentils and **kale** are both bioactive-rich foods that can be paired to address obesity *and* malnutrition around the world. So say Clemson University researchers who think this is possible because the two plants collectively contain most of the bioactive compounds and nutrients required for survival. Going one step further, these researchers evaluated the two based on a food systems approach (all food-related activities involving the production, processing, transport, and consumption of food) and concluded that "brassicas are the perfect complement to pulse crops."[59]

Why? "Because pulses return available nitrogen to the soil, they can improve the yield and nutritional quality of the following (or subsequent) crops. Thus, subsistence farmers would benefit economically from growing pulses and brassica vegetables together through improved soil quality and perhaps even yield; their own diet would also benefit."[60]

Enjoying a plant-based approach and eating plenty of legumes and brassica vegetables can greatly improve the nutritional quality of your diet. The two are a perfect combo for meatless meals such as our Kale and Lentil Super Soup (page 236).

7. WILD-CAUGHT COLD-WATER FISH

Unless you are a vegetarian or vegan, fish is an important protein food to include in your diet. But there are many considerations in selecting the "right" fish. We eat only wild-caught species and avoid farmed fish, which are fed grains and other unnatural ingredients that change their fat makeup. Cold-water fish are rich in omega-3 fats, making their consumption conducive to cardiovascular health. Avoid fish species that are endangered from overfishing. (SeafoodWatch.org provides a list of endangered fish species.) We don't eat bottom-feeders such as shrimp and other shellfish, which are proscribed in the Bible as unclean. For example, shellfish may contain mercury and other toxins such as polychlorinated biphenyl (PCBs), which are injurious to health.

- *Salmon* should be wild and harvested in cold waters, meaning Alaska, the Pacific Northwest, or northern Europe, among other sources. Avoid Atlantic salmon. Omega-3 fatty acids moderate inflammation, so although eating any wild-caught fish addresses inflammation, salmon is one of your best bets.[61,62] In combination with calorie restriction, eating wild salmon has also shown the best results in effecting weight loss and deceasing concentrations of three markers of inflammation.[63]

8. TEAS

Water is the go-to drink in the Essential Oils Diet, but sometimes you need some flavor—that's where tea comes in. Not to mention that herbal teas are chock-full of bioactive compounds. We enjoy a variety of different teas every day.

- *Matcha green tea* is one of the best sources of catechins, bioactive compounds that act as antioxidants. The Japanese have used this powdered form of green tea in tea ceremonies for centuries. Regular consumption offers remarkable healing effects. The National Cancer Institute even acknowledges that it could cure cancer,[64] in part by protecting against damage to DNA. Matcha is also effective at burning body fat.[65] A study of overweight men showed significant fat reduction in those who regularly consumed matcha tea over a twelve-week period, compared with a control group of men who drank none.

  But all green tea is not created equal. A groundbreaking study[66] that used sophisticated technology to determine matcha's chemical makeup found the concentration of a single catechin to be 137 times greater than the amount in China green tips green tea, and at least three times higher than other green teas. Drinking matcha green tea also helps athletes recover after intense workouts and builds cellular strength.[67] Ujido is our favorite brand of matcha, and we often start the day with a matcha latte blended with almond milk (see page 215). Learn more about Ujido and why we love this brand by visiting NaturalLivingFamily.com/ujido.

- *Rooibos and holy basil tea* blends two herbs. Rooibos, which hails from South Africa, contains large amounts of bioactive polyphenolic compounds, and helps you not only to lose pounds but also to achieve your body's ideal weight.[68] Holy basil, known as *tulsi* in India, has been used in Hindu ceremonies since ancient times, hence the "holy" modifier. This Ayurvedic herb increases energy and relieves stress on the body. In combination, the two herbs produce a spicy "warming" tea that can help rev you up when you're feeling sluggish. One of our metabolism-boosting favorites is the Republic of Tea's Get Burning blend, which also includes cordyceps, a medicinal herb used by Chinese athletes to boost energy and endurance, plus the invigorating kick of a little chile pepper.

HONORABLE MENTION

Senna tea has been used for thousands of years to stimulate the intestines, aiding the natural process of elimination. Smooth Move, an herbal blend of senna, fennel, coriander, and ginger, made by Traditional Medicinals, is a natural, gentle bowel cleanser. Best taken at bedtime, it usually works within six to twelve hours.

Get Ready, Get Set

Now that you have an idea of the delicious and proactive foods you'll be eating on the Essential Oils Diet, you'll begin to understand the role that bioactive compounds play in our holistic approach to weight control and overall health. Focus on regularly eating foods from these groups, in moderate portions, of course, and you will be well on your way to achieving your weight-loss goals. We'll get into the specifics in chapter 5.

Review the list of Essential Eight foods and use it to make a shopping list. Then head off to the market so you can hit the ground running after reading the following chapter. Stock up on veggies, fruit, and cold-water fish, and you can get started tomorrow!

the garage if necessary. Again, buy when frozen items are on sale. I don't know how we could eat the way we do without a separate freezer to store our bulk frozen items.

- *Be a biblical (seasonal) shopper.* Buy what's in season, when prices drop. According to Ecclesiastes, "To everything there is a season, and a time to every purpose under Heaven: . . . a time to plant, and a time to pluck up that which is planted." Tomatoes and zucchini are practically given away at the end of summer. The same with berries (even organic ones) in summer. Stock up and freeze or dehydrate what you can't eat over a few days.

- *Buy locally.* Farmers' markets are likely to offer fresher and therefore more nutrient-dense produce than that trucked or flown in. You're also supporting local growers. Wait until just before closing time to get some bargains.

- *Explore online stores.* Thrive Market sells quality products and is cost-effective, especially with free shipping on orders of more than $50. For starters, you can get healthy snacks, shampoo you can feel good about, and toothpaste without sodium lauryl sulfate and other bad ingredients. Amazon is another great option for home-care products. Thrive is giving all new customers who bought this book $20 off their first order. To claim your gift, go to NaturalLivingFamily.com/ThriveMarket.

- *You needn't always opt for organic.* Some conventionally raised produce, such as avocado and pineapple, either has not been as heavily treated with chemicals, or their thick skin or a short growing season minimizes toxins. Save your money and spend it on organic produce that is dramatically safer, such as strawberries and spinach, than the conventional counterpart. See the Dirty Dozen (page 184) and the Clean Fifteen (page 185). On the other hand, if you're going to slurp up smoothies with kale every day, make sure it's organic.

> • *Don't eschew frozen food.* Not everything has to be fresh. If produce is flash-frozen right after being picked, there is minimal nutrient loss. Do avoid canned foods; the BPA (bisphenol A) lining of the can has been shown to be an endocrine disruptor.

To watch a video shopping tour in which Mama Z shows you how she finds great deals on healthy foods at the local grocery store, visit EssentialOilsDiet.com.

Where Should You Start?

The next chapter addresses the Essential Fast Track. To determine whether to start in this phase or go directly to the Essential Lifestyle in chapter 7, ask yourself the following questions:

- *Are you looking to lose weight?* Start with the Fast Track!
- *Are you pleased with your current weight or need to put on a few pounds?* Turn to page 135 to begin with the Essential Lifestyle.
- *Do you have some gastrointestinal issues?* You might benefit from beginning with the Fast Track to uncover whether certain foods are aggravating your condition.

CHAPTER 5

THE 30-DAY ESSENTIAL FAST TRACK: FORM NEW HABITS AND KICK-START WEIGHT LOSS

*"I don't run away from a challenge because I am afraid.
Instead, I run towards it because the only way to
escape fear is to trample it beneath your foot."*
—NADIA COMANECI

Here we go! Time to put into practice everything we have been talking about. And that includes beginning to build new habits that will morph into your transformation. In the Essential Fast Track, you will shed unwanted pounds that are hindering your health, your self-image, your energy level, and even your ability to give your all to your family and others dear to your heart.

Think of the Fast Track as akin to a month of boot camp. It can be hard at times, but when you complete it, you will be incredibly proud of yourself, if not downright dazzled by your resolve. This first phase produces quick results that will encourage you to stay the course.

Dr. Z here. The steps you're going to implement during the next thirty days are somewhat restrictive and are going to require an exceptional amount of self-control. "But the fruit of the Spirit is love, joy, peace, patience, kindness, goodness, faithfulness, gentleness, and *self-control*" (*Galatians 5:22–23*). Whichever path you choose, you're going to need self-control. By doing that and doing it regularly, you get into a much more empowering situation in which this increasingly habitual behavior means that food will not run your life.

The Fast Track, like the Essential Lifestyle that follows, has eight components that work synergistically. (Eight seems to be that special number!) Ideally, you will do all of them from the get-go. But if that is too much, the first four are nonnegotiable. You can then ease into the others.

These are some of the other nonnegotiables if you really want to do the boot camp:

- No smoking
- No alcohol, including wine
- No fruit juice (occasional vegetable juice is okay)
- No dairy
- No conventional grains (wheat, rye, barley, spelt, and such all contain gluten) and no bread (even gluten-free bread)
- No sweets, no sugar, and no artificial sugars (meaning "diet" products). This includes desserts and sweet snacks. Our own desserts are made with natural sugars, but even some of them have too much sugar for Fast Track. As you'll see in the recipes in Part 3, these are indicated with an asterisk after the recipe name. Others may be acceptable if you use stevia rather than a different natural sweetener. Ingredients that may be swapped with stevia are also marked clearly within the recipes.
- No chips, no fried food, and especially no junk food
- No energy drinks, no soda, and no coffee
- No meat or poultry

Note that this is a pure boot camp experience filled with fruits, veggies, legumes, and small portions of ancient grains designed to give you optimal results in the shortest time possible. Beyond those no-no's, as we've said many times, we want to offer you a lot of variety. You'll create your own approach, much like reading a *Choose Your Own Adventure* book, or as we call it, Personalize Your Program. We must remind you that in some cases, the choices you make will impact how quickly you lose weight or how much weight you lose. But, again, it's up to you.

However, if you are struggling through this process, here are some ways that you can continue to see progress *and* satisfy your palate. If your sweet tooth tempts you to fall off the wagon, have a handful of Fill in the Gap Nuts (page 244) or some Essentially Delicious Yogurt (page 229). If either of these won't do the job, have a small portion of Dr. Z's Chocolate-Avocado Puddin' (page 267), Coconut Whipped Cream (page 262), or Mama Z's Vanilla Ice Cream (page 263), with the emphasis on *small*. If your weight loss has stalled, avoid all desserts. You'll see that our sample Fast Track weekly meal plan does not include desserts.

Also, be aware that the various components enhance each other. You will see quicker and better results if you initiate all Eight Essential Habits simultaneously.

To help you get started on the Essential Fast Track, we have compiled an Essential Fast Track Success Package—which includes a starter checklist, shopping guide, and meal plan— that you can download by visiting EssentialOilsDiet.com.

Eight Essential Habits

1. *Consume quality fuel.* Eat lots of vegetables, fruits, nuts, seeds, and legumes—all are packed with bioactive compounds— and if you desire extra protein, stick with wild-caught fish or organic, cage-free eggs. Occasionally enjoying protein-rich grains such as quinoa and millet is okay, but no red meat, poultry, and certainly no pork. (Review the Essential Eight on page 78 for details.) *Personalize Your Program:* If you are a vegan, simply omit any animal products.
2. *Become a body in motion.* Walking at least 2 miles a day and/or

following the program designed by Mama Z (see page 289) is a great way to start. If you already follow an exercise regimen, try to take it to the next level. For more ideas, see Movement: Personalize Your Program on page 105.

3. *Stay well hydrated.* As the Chinese proverb says, "Drinking a daily cup of tea will surely starve the apothecary." Drink plenty of filtered water, herb teas, and matcha green tea (especially if you're a coffee drinker), as well as kombucha and smoothies. We'll discuss this in detail in Proper Hydration: Personalize Your Program on page 107.

4. *Use essential oils.* These help control appetite, increase energy use, and actually melt body fat. Using oils in recipes, as topical applications, and via inhalation are all great options. Best of all, explore all three. Chapter 6 is devoted to their use, and we give you a number of healing remedy options in Part 3.

5. *Fast intermittently.* Give your gut a much-needed break, which is one reason why we advise against consuming red meat, poultry, and pork. You can start by simply eating your last meal of the day by 7 p.m. and enjoying breakfast at least twelve hours later. It's called "break-fast" for a reason, right? For more ideas, see Intermittent Fasting: Personalize Your Program on page 109.

6. *Cleanse your colon.* This will enhance your gastrointestinal tract's ability to assist in weight management. Again, we'll offer several options, including with the use of a gentle herbal tea you drink before bed. For more ideas, see Cleanse Your Colon: Personalize Your Program on page 111.

7. *Get plenty of shut-eye.* Sleep plays a significant role in weight loss, and using essential oils will be a game-changer in helping you fall asleep and stay asleep! See A Good Night's Sleep: Personalize Your Program on page 112.

8. *Spend some time in the sun.* If possible, get at least twenty minutes of sun exposure every day. If you live in a climate where this is not possible, supplement with vitamin D. See Sunlight: Personalize Your Program on page 113 to explore some alternatives.

Ancient Antecedents

Eating this way is hardly new. You could think of it as a Garden of Eden lifestyle, in which God provides what we need to thrive. Consuming meat occasionally and avoiding it at other times both have antecedents in the Old Testament. Fasting is an essential component of most spiritual practices. And as prescribed in the Bible, the Quran, and other sacred texts, we do not recommend eating pork or shellfish as these foods have traditionally been considered unclean and therefore potentially dangerous and inherently unhealthful.

Along with regular physical activity and the use of essential oils—which we will discuss in detail in chapter 6—you will be incorporating another habit that may or may not be familiar to you: regular colon cleansing. Before you say "yuck," read why these practices are key to good health and weight management in the following chapters. We'll also give you a number of fasting and cleansing options so you can pick those with which you feel most comfortable. Now, let's discuss the Eight Essential Habits in more detail.

1. QUALITY FUEL: PERSONALIZE YOUR PROGRAM

This is the most important piece of the Fast Track, so we'll park here for a while before discussing the other seven Essential Habits.

The Essential Oils Diet excludes very few foods, among them processed sugar, pork, and shellfish. Other items, such as dairy and bread, don't belong on the Fast Track when you will be shedding most of your excess weight but can be reintroduced when you move to the Essential Lifestyle. Also off the menu for now is coffee, which can cause stomach distress, to say nothing of potentially interfering with sufficient sleep, which you now know is essential for weight loss. Finally, you'll avoid alcohol, a known factor for obesity,[7] for the time being.

Our premise in restricting certain foods and recommending others (i.e., the Essential Eight in chapter 4) during the Fast Track is to boost your natural fat-burning capacity, help you regain control of your palate, and put you in the driver's seat.

There's no right or wrong way to do this program, but these are the concepts you need to buy into. You've got to find what works for you, which includes coming up with your own daily meal plans. We think you'll be more successful if you create meal plans from recipes you love and enjoy preparing, but if you prefer to be told exactly what to eat, we've also provided a Fast Track–approved sample meal plan that you can follow to the letter.

Here are some other tips:

- Not sure what to eat for breakfast? Whole fruit and vegetable smoothies are always a good option! Eggs are fine on the Fast Track, and if you want to maximize weight loss, have egg-white veggie omelets instead of whole eggs or smoothies.
- Dithering about what to eat for lunch? You can't go wrong with a big salad!

- Not sure what to snack on? Nuts and seeds do the trick!
- Wondering what to have for dinner? Beans or lentils fill you up and provide ample nutrition when mixed with cruciferous veggies!

Dinner is where you can have some fun. Be sure to try some of Mama Z's delicious recipes in Part 3. These are our easy-to-prepare, go-to recipes for both phases of the program. On page 100 is a blank meal plan to scan and print out. A sample weekly meal plan follows to show how to use the Fast Track recipes to construct your own meals (and you can also use this exact meal plan instead of coming up with your own, if you prefer!). We suggest you post your meal plan somewhere in the kitchen where it's highly visible and use it to help make up your grocery shopping list.

Note: If you're trying to lose extra weight, limit your breakfast to drinking Living Fuel SuperGreens. Simply add 1 to 2 scoops of the powder to 24 ounces of purified water and mix in a blender bottle. If you need an early morning or midday pick-me-up, make the Fat-Burning Matcha Latte (page 215) to give you that extra boost. Many coffee shops now have matcha on their menus, so you can get one on the go as long as they have unsweetened almond or coconut milk.

Here are some additional tips you'll find helpful:

- *Sweet stuff.* Avoid any form of sugar. This includes processed sugar, meaning white sugar, brown sugar, confectioners' sugar, and so on. All are off the menu for good. In Fast Track, you'll also omit all natural sweeteners that are not included in the approved meal plan recipes: coconut sugar (aka coconut crystals), honey or honey crystals, maple syrup (preferably Grade B—now called Grade A Dark or Grade C), molasses, and monk fruit. Having said that, a scant teaspoon of honey in your morning cuppa tea is fine. There is also a smidgen of honey in Mama Z's recipe for Fill in the Gap Nuts (page 244). Xylitol, erythritol, and other sugar alcohols are also acceptable, but do understand that they can cause digestive problems, including gassiness and diarrhea, if

7-DAY ESSENTIAL FAST TRACK MEAL PLAN

	Breakfast	Lunch	Dinner	Snack/Dessert
Monday				
Tuesday				
Wednesday				
Thursday				
Friday				
Saturday				
Sunday				

7-DAY ESSENTIAL FAST TRACK MEAL PLAN

	Breakfast	Lunch	Dinner	Snack/Dessert
Monday	Water or vegetable juice fast or **Greens and Herb Omelet** (page 222)	**Avocado Egg Salad** (page 226) on greens	**Kale and Lentil Super Soup** (page 236) and side garden salad	**Fill in the Gap Nuts** (page 244)
Tuesday	**Berry Green Delight Smoothie** (page 224) or Living Fuel SuperGreens	**Greens and Herb Omelet** (page 222)	**Mama Z's Spaghetti** (page 249) over spinach	**Mama Z's Hummus** (page 242) with fresh-cut veggies for dipping
Wednesday	**Cacao Energy Bowl** (page 224) or Living Fuel SuperGreens	**Avocado Egg Salad** (page 226) on greens	**Slow-Cooker Lasagna** (page 248) made with eggplant or zucchini strips	**Fill in the Gap Nuts** (page 244)
Thursday	**Greens and Herb Omelet** (page 222) or Living Fuel SuperGreens	**Kale and Lentil Super Soup** (page 236)	**South of the Border Casserole** (page 252) and side garden salad	**Mama Z's Hummus** (page 242) and fresh-cut veggies for dipping
Friday	**Mama Z's Bioactive Breakfast Shake** (page 222) or Living Fuel SuperGreens	**Tasty Tomato Bisque** (page 235)	Poached or grilled wild-caught salmon and **Mama Z's Coleslaw** (page 230)	**Fill in the Gap Nuts** (page 244)
Saturday	**Nutty Chocolate Protein Smoothie** (page 223) or Living Fuel SuperGreens	**Mama Z's Coleslaw** (page 230) and hard-boiled eggs	**Garden-Fresh Quinoa Salad** (page 251)	Half a Hass avocado with a dollop of **Mama Z's Hummus** (page 242)
Sunday	**Essentially Delicious Yogurt** (page 229) or Living Fuel SuperGreens	**Tasty Tomato Bisque** (page 235)	**Bok Choy Super Stir-Fry** (page 245) over Miracle Noodles	**Fill in the Gap Nuts** (page 244)

consumed in excess.[8] The jury is still out on agave nectar, so we advise steering clear of it. The natural sugar in fresh fruit is also fine.

- *Grain alert.* Again, no conventional grains (wheat, barley, rye, spelt, etc.)—all contain gluten—or bread (even gluten-free bread) are permitted while on the Essential Fast Track. Ancient grains are okay in small portions as you'll see in the meal plan on page 101. Brown rice, quinoa, millet, and other nutrient-rich ancient grains are fine only if you follow the approved recipes in the Essential Fast Track Meal Plan because they incorporate very small portions. You can reintroduce ancient grains without restriction in the Essential Lifestyle, but continue to avoid any genetically modified grains.

  Organic grains are inherently non-GMO, but conventionally grown grains, particularly wheat, which are almost always GMO, remain off-limits for good.

- *Seriously, no coffee.* Yes, we understand that coffee is rich in polyphenols and other such bioactive compounds. And, yes, we know that coffee has been shown to help improve glucose tolerance and slow down weight gain in studies with mice.[9,10] Still we request that you steer clear of joe during the Fast Track.

  Why? Primarily because coffee is highly addictive (physically, emotionally, and psychologically), and this one-month journey is all about regaining control of your life.[11] We also needn't remind you that coffee is acidic. It's also a diuretic. Drinking matcha green tea is infinitely more beneficial in almost every way.

  You can resume drinking the occasional cup of coffee in the Essential Lifestyle phase, though don't be surprised if you fail to fall back into old habits. Our observation is that most people do not go back to their daily cuppa (or three) after the Fast Track. We hope that this is the case for you because a *high dose of caffeine* (i.e., just three 8-ounce cups of coffee a day) promotes acid reflux[12] and is a known sleep disruptor.[13]

- *Tubers.* In addition to the Essential Eight—our favorite and best-researched foods (see page 78)—tubers are great alternatives to grains to round out a meal. Sweet potatoes, white potatoes, cassava, yams, and yucca are just some of the many tubers out there, although there are others not yet common in this country.

  But, with the exception of sweet potatoes, tubers are too starchy to eat in the Fast Track. On the other hand, if you need to put on some pounds, starchy but healthy carbohydrates can help, so any kind of tuber belongs in your grocery cart. They all are full of fiber and other bioactive compounds and come in a rainbow of colors. Sweet potatoes boast a host of flavonoids, such as beta-carotene, a powerful natural antioxidant. These are all good reasons to consume them, but here's a new twist. According to a Japanese study, consuming the starchy water in which sweet potatoes have been cooked may help digestion and weight loss![14]

- *Eating out.* Because of poor options plus the preservatives and chemicals found in most restaurants, we recommend you limit eating out in the Fast Track phase. If you travel a lot, are required to go to social events, or just don't have time to prepare all of your meals—been there, done that—choose your restaurants wisely. Be sure to stay away from anything lathered in sauces—they are filled with preservatives, sodium, and other chemicals.

  A safe bet would be a dinner salad with grilled wild-caught fish (a good source of healthy omega-3s) and some steamed veggies on the side. If baked sweet potato is an option, choose that and sprinkle it with a little bit of stevia. It'll fill you up and satisfy your craving for sweet things so you won't be tempted to order dessert!

In chapter 7 we offer more advice on how to eat out, manage social events, and stay on course while traveling and in special circumstances such as when your kids leave the nest for college.

Before you begin your own makeover, you'll want to make over your kitchen by removing foods that you will find especially tempting. Instead of tossing food out, please inquire if your house of worship collects food for the needy or if you can give it to a homeless shelter or another organization that helps those in need.

THE IMPORTANCE OF HEALTHY MEAL REPLACEMENTS

When we are fasting, trying to trim up and slim down for a special event such as a reunion or a beauty pageant, or when we simply want an extra boost of bioactive-powered nutrition, we turn to Living Fuel, which is a super meal that you can literally drink. (Mama Z's Super Greens Powder or Super Reds Powder is full of nutrients but is not a complete meal replacement.) There are very few of these products you can use with confidence, and Ensure is definitely not one of them.

Our dear friend K. C. Craichy developed Living Fuel more than sixteen years ago to deal with his wife's serious nutritional deficiencies and resultant health problems. Today, she has never been healthier. Living Fuel is a gluten-free, all-natural, greens-based whole meal superfood that provides all of your daily nutritional requirements and more in one delicious super smoothie. No other greens product even comes close to matching its nutritional profile.

If you're trying to lose extra weight during the Essential Fast Track, drink Living Fuel every morning for breakfast—and for lunch, too. Simply add 1 to 2 scoops of Living Fuel SuperGreens or SuperBerry powder to 24 ounces of purified water and mix in a blender bottle. If you're happy with your weight, adding either to your favorite shakes, smoothies, and acai bowls is an ideal way to boost your nutritional profile. Just add one scoop and you're good to go. To learn more about Living Fuel, visit NaturalLivingFamily .com/LivingFuel.

NO, IT'S NOT MORE EXPENSIVE

When you eat healthy, you'll save a lot of money. We're serious!

Junk food isn't satisfying, so the effects aren't lasting. Eating a salad, on the other hand, will keep you going for a couple hours or more. Have a burger and you'll get fatigued and then want to eat another one soon after. It's a vicious cycle that obese people battle.

Healthy snacks such as a baked sweet potato or grilled Brussels sprouts can be meals themselves. Plus they're cheap and easy to make. Hands down, if you make the majority of your own food with organic, non-GMO ingredients, it will save you money in the long run.

There are no shortcuts, but there are time-savers you can employ in following this lifestyle. When it comes to life, you are going to pay either on the front end or the back end. If you eat the fast-paced-lifestyle way, you're more likely to gain weight and have attendant health problems. So even though that kind of food appears to be less expensive in the short run, you are going to end up paying way more because you'll be eating more and your medical bills will be through the roof!

2. MOVEMENT: PERSONALIZE YOUR PROGRAM

Why must you exercise if you are cutting down on your food intake and eating a better diet? We thought you'd never ask! For starters, regular exercise tones your body so you look slimmer and your clothes fit better, even if your weight is unchanged. But regular movement, and particularly high-intensity interval training (HIIT), offers numerous other benefits:

- Boosting your energy level by taking in more oxygen[15]
- Enhancing your metabolism so you burn more calories even at rest[16]
- Reducing insulin resistance, particularly via vigorous-intensity exercise training[17,18]

- Building muscle tissue, which burns more calories than fat tissue does[19]
- Improving bone density—especially in older adults[20]
- Increasing emotional intelligence (the awareness of how you feel) and regulating mood[21]

If you currently don't exercise or have gotten out of the habit, choose a few of the low-impact exercises Mama Z recommends (see page 289) to target key muscle groups. Do them regularly, increasing the number of sets and reps over time.

Here are some other tips.

- If you already have a walking or jogging routine, consider finding a partner or joining a club. If you know people are waiting for you, you'll be motivated to get out there every day.
- If you already exercise or walk regularly, consider increasing your daily mileage and/or adding some of the exercises on page 293 to your usual routine, all of which you can do at home without having to buy any expensive gear.
- Sign up for exercise classes. We're big fans of group fitness, especially the HIIT you can find at Orangetheory (OrangeTheoryFitness.com) and similar studios nationwide. Working out with others produces a kind of energy that helps you push yourself to heights you might not reach alone.
- Working with a personal trainer is always a good idea and can be a great gift to yourself. A trainer will assess your current level of fitness and tailor a program to your needs. He or she will also make sure you are doing individual moves properly so as not to cause injury or strain.

The point is that you can customize your movement and fitness program to suit your budget, your level of fitness, and your goals. Find what works for you and make it fun so you can stick with it! And be sure to add your fitness goals and progress to your Transformation Journal.

WALK AS THOUGH YOUR LIFE DEPENDS ON IT

If you haven't heard, sitting is the new smoking.

Sitting for excessively long periods of time is a risk factor for early death, per a 2017 study published in *Annals of Internal Medicine*.[22] "Sit less, move more" is the American Heart Association's advice.[23] Here are some practical ways to make movement a way of life:

- If you have a desk job, make a point of standing part of the time instead of staying glued to your chair. Take a short break every hour or so. Do squats while on conference calls. Walk to the water cooler and back. Go outside to get some fresh air. Take the stairs instead of an elevator or escalator whenever you can.
- Instead of meeting a friend for lunch, take a walk together.
- Use a pedometer, a Fitbit, or an app on your smartphone to track the number of steps or miles you walk each day to motivate yourself. Don't forget to record each day's number in your journal.
- When shopping, park your car at the far end of the lot.
- Choose your friends wisely. If your social activities center on exercise and movement-type activities, you'll be better served than going to a bar or sitting in a movie theater.

3. PROPER HYDRATION: PERSONALIZE YOUR PROGRAM

Drinking several glasses of water throughout the day is a good habit to prevent dehydration, which often causes hunger pangs that will lead you to overeat. Dehydration has also been linked to low cognitive and athletic performance and poor gastrointestinal function, as well as headaches and heart problems.[24]

On the flip side, drinking too much water can cause bloating, can dilute your stomach acid—hindering your digestion—and can give you an unnatural feeling of fullness that can backfire with binge eating when hunger pangs hit at night!

This is important to consider because the jury is still out on whether or not increased water consumption can help you lose weight.[25] Instead, the type of water you drink, not the amount, seems to have the most impact. Drinking 16 ounces (500 ml) of water, for example, was found to increase metabolic rate by 30 percent.[26] However, heating water from 22°C to 37°C (71.6°F to 98.6°F) accounted for 40 percent of this change.

Finding the right hydration set point, therefore, is just as critical as knowing when to stop eating. Just as you will be learning how to eat until you are 80 percent full (see No Need to Count Anything on page 70 for a refresher), pay close attention to your body and drink when you need to.

If you're not sure whether you need to rehydrate, test your skin turgor, or elasticity. The National Institutes of Health–sponsored MedlinePlus explains that you can test your skin turgor by simply pinching the skin on the back of your hand for a few seconds. If your skin immediately returns to normal, you are hydrated. If it doesn't, you need to drink up.[27]

Find plain water boring or off in taste? These alternatives can make it easy to stay hydrated:

- Instead of buying some fancy "designer water," make your own herb- or fruit-infused water by simply putting some mint, lemongrass, and/or other herbs into a glass jar. Add fresh melon chunks, lemon slices, or berries and water and let it sit in the fridge overnight. Delish!
- Drink matcha tea (see page 215).
- Drink hot or iced herb tea—explore organic mint, ginger, rooibos, and chamomile, for starters—sweetened with stevia if you wish.
- Try kombucha tea, which is made from a fermented symbiotic culture of healthful probiotic bacteria and yeast—SCOBY for short. It is a natural antibiotic packed with vitamins and antioxidants that boost your immune system and aid digestion as it hydrates your body.

Place one drop of lime essential oil and some liquid stevia extract in a 32-ounce glass bottle and fill with sparkling water to sip throughout the day. The fizziness helps you feel satiated and the lime oil assists in fat-burning.

4. AROMATHERAPY: PERSONALIZE YOUR PROGRAM

How often have your efforts to slim down been derailed by uncontrollable cravings for the very foods you know you should avoid? Or are you often so hungry that when mealtime rolls around you can't control your appetite? Essential oils to the rescue!

Grapefruit, lime, cinnamon, and peppermint are our go-to weight-loss oils. Inhaling grapefruit essential oil has been shown to decrease your appetite and stimulate the breakdown of fats, called lipolysis, as well as thermogenesis, the burning of calories for body heat.[28] In chapter 6, we will get into greater detail about these oils, as well as others that can indirectly impact weight loss.

5. INTERMITTENT FASTING: PERSONALIZE YOUR PROGRAM

Intermittent fasting is simply electing not to eat at certain times, which could be a matter of hours or last up to a day or more—without necessarily reducing your overall intake. Whether you realize it or not, you are fasting every day, or every night more accurately. Unless you have a midnight snack, you fast from the end of dinner until breakfast the following day. Conscious fasting is optional, but we have to say that nothing clears the body—and the mind—better than giving your digestive system a break for half a day or more. You may want to make intermittent fasting a daily or weekly habit or opt for any other time frame.

As with most aspects of the Essential Oils Diet, you create your own program. Our preference would be for you to initiate the Fast

Track with a twenty-four-hour water fast. But here are other ways to fast.

- Do a shorter water fast.
- Drink only liquids such as a Living Fuel shake or Mama Z's Bioactive Breakfast Shake (page 222), kombucha, herb teas, and/or even some vegetable juice for a day.
- Have a single meal in a twenty-four-hour period, perhaps eating dinner and then not eating again until the same time the next day. This allows you to go to bed satiated and sleep for a good part of the fast.
- Simply skip one meal—for example, going from an early dinner one day to lunch the following day, meaning you fast for sixteen hours or so.
- Go vegan for twenty-four hours, eating just fruits and veggies.

Any fast is restrictive, but you could start with those lower on the list and work up to a water fast. The health benefits of fasting include burning fat and healing the gut,[29] and it also offers a spiritual dimension via the humble mind-set of giving up something to get closer to God.

There are also significant spiritual benefits to fasting, which is a component of most faiths. We encourage you—even challenge you—to give it a try, even if you decide to skip just one meal. Whether you are Jewish, Buddhist, Muslim, or Hindu, or if you follow a New Age philosophy, you can adopt these principles and cleanse your body as you simultaneously let it be a time when you ask people to forgive you or make something you've done wrong, right.

Potential trouble signs include difficulty sleeping, hair loss, low energy during the day, menstrual irregularity, irritability, light-headedness or dizziness, and extreme weight loss or inexplicable weight gain. Pay attention to your body's cues as you attempt inter-mittent fasting. You may be one of the people for whom it works, or you may need to alter your habits to apply the principles in another way. As always, seek only the best for your body and life.

6. CLEANSE YOUR COLON:
PERSONALIZE YOUR PROGRAM

Ideally, you want to clean out your system before you begin the Essential Fast Track. This may be a delicate subject, but cleaning out your colon can help speed weight loss and eliminate toxins from your system, especially if you're not having regular bowel movements (that is, at least once or twice a day). Unfortunately, because of the lack of evidence evaluating the effects of colon hydrotherapy (aka colonics) and enemas on the body, the medical community generally recommends against them.[31]

Our personal experience suggests otherwise. The testimonials we've received from the people to whom we have recommended both procedures have been nothing less than fantastic, including such positive reactions as increased energy, bowel regularity, pain reduction, and weight loss. If you have concerns, consult with your health-care provider before doing an enema or colonic.

There are several ways to go—pun intended!

- Colon hydrotherapy is a great means to do this. We recommend getting one the weekend before you start the Fast Track, then follow your colon hydrotherapist's recommendation on how to proceed during the following month.

- Try an enema.
- Do a saltwater flush: First thing in the morning, dissolve 2 tablespoons of noniodized sea salt in 32 ounces of warm water, then drink it all at once. It usually takes about an hour to flush out your system, so stay near the bathroom!
- Add more fiber to your diet in the form of psyllium husks to bulk your stool, encouraging regular bowel movements.
- Drink a cup of Traditional Medicinal's Smooth Move tea before bed. This gentle laxative delivers reliable results the next morning.

7. A GOOD NIGHT'S SLEEP: PERSONALIZE YOUR PROGRAM

Did you know that 35 percent of Americans average less than seven hours of nightly shut-eye,[32] the minimum amount adults need to function optimally? Sleep is essential to allow your brain and your body to hit the reset button, eliminating toxins and restoring cells, which also acts as a brake on the aging process.[33,34]

And are you aware that lack of sleep is implicated as a cause of being overweight? A sixteen-year longitudinal study of about sixty thousand nurses, all of whom were initially healthy and not obese, found that over the course of the study, those who slept five hours or less a night had a 15 percent greater chance of becoming obese and a 30 percent greater chance of gaining thirty pounds than women who regularly got seven hours of sleep.[35,36] Many factors are at play. Sleep deprivation disrupts the balance of certain hormones that control appetite. Moreover, being tired reduces the incentive to exercise, and the longer a person is awake, the more opportunities they have to eat.

Your first order of business is to get more sleep, but this is easier said than done, depending on your work schedule and family responsibilities. If that is not possible, you can certainly improve the quality of your sleep by minimizing common sleep disturbances as much as possible. Try these suggestions on for size:

- Set a regular lights-out time.
- Establish a bedtime routine that allows you to unwind.
- Don't eat late at night or drink caffeinated beverages after 5 p.m.
- Keep your bedroom dark and turn off any electronic devices in the room that emit blue light, which interferes with sleep. That means your TV, cell phone, and Wi-Fi router.
- Yoga or another form of gentle exercise an hour or so before bed helps regulate serotonin, the hormone that helps you relax and sleep better.[37]
- Inhale or diffuse lavender or other relaxing essential oils at bedtime. Numerous research studies[38,39,40] support lavender's ability to relieve symptoms such as sleep disturbance and anxiety, without the side effects associated with over-the-counter or prescribed drugs.[41]
- Finally, buy the best mattress you can afford. You spend a third of your life on it! We like the Sleep Number bed.

8. SUNLIGHT: PERSONALIZE YOUR PROGRAM

One hundred years ago people regularly spent time outdoors, but no more. As a result, vitamin D deficiency has become epidemic, with numerous health implications, including compromised bone density and weight gain.[42,43] Although most people are not severely deficient in this nutrient, "subclinical" deficiency, meaning lower-than-normal vitamin D levels without visible signs or symptoms, is common. Your body makes vitamin D when your skin is exposed to direct sunlight. You have various options to get sufficient vitamin D:

- Spend at least twenty minutes, and better yet half an hour, a day in the sun, preferably before noon. This habit also sets your circadian rhythm, or biological clock, making it easier for you to fall asleep at night. People who get their dose of sunshine earlier in the day have been shown to have a lower BMI than those who get exposure in the afternoon.[44]

- Vitamin D is also found in such foods as cheese made from the milk of grass-fed cattle and sheep, as well as in wild-caught cold-water fish. Eat wild-caught salmon and other fatty fish regularly.
- If you want to take a supplement, keep in mind that recent evidence supports that combining vitamins D and K is more effective than taking either alone for bone and cardiovascular health.[45]
- We like to take a supplement that combines 2,500 IU of vitamin D_3 plus 100 mcg of vitamin K_2 during the winter months when we don't get a lot of sun exposure.

What's Next?

Once you have achieved your goal weight—or close to it—or thirty days are up, you are well on your way to developing new habits and beginning to transform yourself. You can now move to the less-restrictive Essential Lifestyle. However, if you still have more weight to lose and believe you can continue to handle boot camp longer, stay here. And once you have said goodbye to those pesky extra pounds, understand that making the Essential Lifestyle permanent is the key to your commitment to maintaining a healthy weight and overall wellness.

Before we dive into this lifetime "phase," turn the page to explore how to use essential oils to help you reach your weight-loss goal.

CHAPTER 6

ESSENTIAL OILS FOR WEIGHT-LOSS SUPPORT

"Never go to a doctor whose office plants have died."
—ERMA BOMBECK

In this chapter we will set the record straight on the benefits of using essential oils for weight loss. We will break down the research that tells us which oils are effective (and which ones you may want to steer away from) and also set the groundwork so that you can start to make and use the aromatherapy recipes in Part 3 with confidence!

But, before we do so, we need to discuss some key safety considerations because essential oils are potent plant-based bioactive compounds and can have a powerful effect on your body.

Safety First

Your skin soaks up chemicals like a sponge, so you need to be extremely careful about what you put on it. (The same goes for what you put *in* your body.) Even though essential oils are bioactive compounds, these highly concentrated ingredients can interact with your skin, possibly causing an allergic response or contact dermatitis (also known as sensitization).

This is not to scare you away from using essential oils. They are actually at the bottom of the list of chemicals that can cause reactions with overexposure. Believe it or not, it is safer to use essential oils than to plunge into a chlorinated swimming pool.[1] Still, your body is not designed to have these oils slathered on "neat." Rather, you need to dilute them with what is called a carrier oil.

Trust us, friends don't let friends use essential oils neat. As a general rule of thumb, you will use three drops of essential oils to each tablespoon of carrier oil in topical applications. If you have particularly sensitive skin, you might want to start with half that much essential oil. The dilution chart below provides further guidelines.

Proper dilution is essential, with ratio the key. For a roller bottle, the typical dilution for an adult is 2 percent essential oil to the amount of carrier oil. Start with this level of dilution, following the chart below.

ROLLER BOTTLE DILUTION GUIDE

Since roller bottles usually come in 5-, 10-, or 15-milliliter bottles, the standard conversions in Chapter 2 won't apply. Here is a simple dilution guide to get you started for those quantities.

	5-ML ROLLER BOTTLE (1 TEASPOON)	10-ML ROLLER BOTTLE (2 TEASPOONS)
0.5%	Less than 1 drop	1 drop
1.0%	1.5 drops	3 drops
2.0%	3 drops	6 drops
3.0%	4.5 drops	9 drops
4.0%	6 drops	12 drops
5.0%	7.5 drops	15 drops

Two-for-One Benefit

Many of the topical remedy recipes we share in Part 3 call for carrier oils. It's important to choose the right one(s) to help you reach your health goals.

Carrier oils are fatty extracts, usually cold-pressed from such sources as almonds, olives, and coconuts, that make an excellent medium to disperse the more concentrated essential oil across your skin. Unlike essential oils, carrier oils are nutritive. They also have healing properties of their own, such as being soothing and anti-inflammatory.

Easy Kitchen Carrier Oils

Before you run out and buy a bunch of different kinds of carrier oils, we suggest you start in your kitchen, where you may already have both olive oil and coconut oil. Both are relatively thick, making them useful as an emollient, as well as for culinary preparations.

- *Olive oil.* Your food can be medicine, literally. Olive oil is exceptionally healing and has actually been proven to help heal foot ulcers![2] Your best bet is extra-virgin olive oil, which is extracted with cold-pressing, rather than heat or chemicals.
- *Coconut oil.* This saturated oil is creamy or solid rather than liquid at room temperature. It penetrates the skin nicely but does tend to leave a slightly greasy residue. Like olive oil, coconut oil heals wounds, presumably by increasing the body's antioxidant levels after being applied to the skin.[3]

   Cold-pressed coconut oil is processed at temperatures that never exceed 120°F, while expeller-pressed coconut oil is processed at temperatures that never exceed 210°F. Higher temperatures reduce the nutritional value.
- *Fractionated coconut oil (FCO).* A process that removes long-chain fatty acids renders FCO always liquid, making it ideal for roller bottle recipes. Unlike regular coconut oil, FCO will not harden, doesn't leave any residue on your skin, and will never get rancid, extending the shelf life of essential oil blends and making it cost-effective.

Popular Nut and Seed Carrier Oils

Packed with vitamins A and E and other nutrients, nut and seed oils are useful for lotions and in roller bottles. *Warning:* If you are allergic to nut oils, stay away from both almond and jojoba oils and use avocado, olive, or grapeseed oil instead.

- *Almond oil.* This mildly scented and flavored oil is both nutrient rich and versatile, known to improve complexion and skin tone.[4] Again, if you're allergic to tree nuts, steer clear of it.
- *Jojoba oil.* With a thicker consistency than almond oil, jojoba is able to penetrate deep into the skin and cells and deliver powerful anti-inflammatory effects.[5] A long shelf life makes it handy for small dilution preparations. Once more, avoid jojoba if you are allergic to nuts.

Fruit Seed Carrier Oils

Extracted from the seeds of fruits, these oils are especially effective for deep hydration, making them ideal for massage oils as well as lip and body balms. More expensive than other carrier oils, fruit seed oils can be found in health food stores and most well-stocked grocery stores, although you can also order them online. These are some of the more common oils:

- *Apricot oil.* Available as expeller-pressed or cold-pressed, the difference is simply one of texture and preference. (Again, cold-pressed oils are processed at lower temperatures than expeller-pressed oils.) Apricot oil's nutrient profile includes vitamins E and A, or at least the carotenoid precursor to vitamin A. It is edible as well as beneficial topically.[6] Because it is both incredibly gentle and nourishing, apricot oil is a good choice for applications that will cover a good deal of skin or that will be heavily applied to children.

- *Avocado oil.* Made from the smooth flesh around the pit, avocado oil is exceptionally rich in nutrients, as is the fruit. An emollient, the oil is excellent for nourishing dry, damaged, or chapped skin.[7]
- *Grapeseed oil.* Another common culinary oil, grapeseed contains high levels of beneficial fatty acids and antioxidants.[8] A relatively light oil, it leaves less of a greasy film on skin than more saturated oils.

Essential Fatty Acid Carrier Oils

Although most of the carrier oils we've discussed thus far are decent sources of essential fatty acids, some oils are considered more robust sources of these vital nutrients. Rich in fatty acid gamma-linolenic acid (GLA), borage and primrose top the list of such carrier oils.

- *Borage oil.* Made from the seeds of a perennial herb, borage oil is an excellent source of gamma-linolenic acid, an anti-inflammatory omega-6 fatty acid. It is widely used as a nutritional supplement and topically for such skin conditions as dermatitis.[9]
- *Evening primrose oil.* Named for the flower that opens only in the evening, evening primrose oil is delicate, so it should be stored in the refrigerator and not added to any heated preparations. It has traditionally been used for women's health and been clinically shown to reduce menopausal hot flashes.[10]

The Power of Scent

Okay, now that you know more about safety and which carrier oils are best to use, let's switch gears to see how essential oils can help you reach your weight-loss goals. Trust us, it's not hocus-pocus. There is an entire branch of science that validates why essential oils "work."

Scent can communicate to your body that it's time to burn fat. According to one study, "Olfactory stimulation with scent of grapefruit oil excites the sympathetic nerve innervating the white adipose [fat] tissue. It [the scent] can also reduce appetite and body weight."[11] Pretty cool, huh? But let's go a little deeper.

Inhaling volatile organic compounds has a direct effect not just on your body but also on your brain. That's because these compounds affect the limbic system of your brain (aka your primal brain) that controls emotions, mood, and memory. This explains why certain scents can be associated with certain memories and can even trigger post-traumatic stress.

Here's how it works: When you smell a rose, for example, the volatile organic compounds in the rose oil dissolve in the mucous lining on the roof of your nasal cavity and stimulate olfactory receptors. Sensory neurons carry signals from your receptors to your brain's olfactory bulb, which filters and then processes the input signals of the rose scent. Next, mitral cells carry output signals to the olfactory cortex, which allows you to perceive and recognize the rose scent. This system is amazingly complex, but even more amazing is that it happens within an instant.

The Limbic Brain and Your Weight

What role does the limbic brain play in weight management? In simple terms, the scents of various essential oils impact your brain's responses. A response to grapefruit oil can decrease your appetite and even stimulate fat breakdown. Orange oil can help alleviate depression, making you less likely to reach for (junk) food to cheer you up. Peppermint oil boosts your energy level by relaxing bronchial smooth muscles, thereby expanding your lung capacity so you can breathe in more oxygen. The result is that your cells burn fat more efficiently.[12]

Alone or in combination, essential oils offer stimulating, appetite-curbing benefits that can be used when cravings hit, at mealtime, or when working out. Essential oils also come into play in addressing health issues that can impact weight management. For example, cinnamon oil can improve glycemic control and provide some protection to the pancreas, enhancing insulin regulation. Both of these factors are crucial for diabetics and helpful for anyone to better manage excess glucose, rather than store it as body fat.

But we're not done yet. Candida overgrowth, inflammation, insufficient or poor sleep, stress, depression, and hormone imbalance can all sabotage your weight-loss and weight-maintenance efforts. (Some of these conditions, along with cancer and other diseases, also make it difficult to *maintain* a healthy weight.) Happily, they, too, can all be addressed with essential oil therapies. Finally, and more importantly, essential oils can be beneficial in dealing with gut issues, which can also sabotage slimming efforts. We'll look more closely at the most helpful essential oils for such conditions.

The Big Four

Now, what you've been waiting for! Let's take a closer look at the four essential oils most effective in supporting appetite reduction, fat-burning, and other processes key to weight loss: grapefruit, lime, peppermint, and cinnamon. The efficacy and properties of this quartet are also best supported by research. All can be used in recipes and for topical applications, diffusion, and inhalation.

1. GRAPEFRUIT ESSENTIAL OIL

You've undoubtedly seen grapefruit recommended as a weight-loss food. No wonder: Every part of the grapefruit, right down to the essential oil in its rind, is good for your metabolism and body composition.

Grapefruit oil and other citrus oils have similar properties: all contain a phytochemical known as d-limonene, which is also found in dillseed, caraway seed, and silver fir needle oil. One study discovered that inhaling grapefruit essential oil decreases food intake, can literally stimulate fat breakdown (known as lipolysis), and simultaneously encourages thermogenesis, the burning of calories to produce body heat.[13] Just inhaling grapefruit oil for fifteen minutes, three times a week, has been shown to control unhealthy food cravings and curb hunger, reducing food intake and body weight.[14]

Topical applications that include grapefruit oil, such as in a massage oil, are also beneficial for weight reduction. In one study, postmenopausal women who regularly massaged their abdomen for six weeks with a combination of grapefruit and cypress essential oils (in a 3 percent solution) showed a decrease in tummy fat, waist size, and cellulite, along with significantly increased self-esteem.[15]

Try for Yourself: Massage Mama Z's Fat-Burning Roll-On blend (page 275) of grapefruit and five other essential oils on your tummy and thighs. She used this combination when preparing for the 2017 and 2018 Mrs. Georgia America pageants. In the most recent event, she won the swimsuit competition (after having four children!) and snagged the first runner-up spot as well.

2. LIME ESSENTIAL OIL

D-limonene is also credited for lime's ability to naturally suppress appetite, promote weight loss, and prevent weight gain.[16] This powerful chemical found in the rind of all citrus fruits possesses many other therapeutic properties, among them acting as an anti-inflammatory.[17,18] Again, inflammation can interfere with weight loss. In addition to containing a copious amount of weight loss–promoting d-limonene, lime oil can also profoundly decrease stress, which can result in overeating, specifically eating junk foods.

Completely safe to consume, lime oil is a tasty weight-loss hack that you can easily add to many of your favorite food items. Simply add a drop per serving to your coconut milk yogurt, guacamole, or stevia-sweetened sparkling water.

Another best practice to harness the fat-burning properties of lime essential oil is to diffuse a fat-burning blend shortly before eating a meal. We like adding grapefruit, cinnamon, and peppermint to lime oil for a true aromatic—and fat-burning—treat!

Try for Yourself: Make a 2 percent dilution by mixing three drops each of cinnamon, grapefruit, lime, and peppermint essential oils in a small glass container with 1 ounce (6 teaspoons) of jojoba oil. Then rub it into the back of your neck and abdomen, which produces a systemic effect as essential oils reach the bloodstream within minutes.

3. PEPPERMINT ESSENTIAL OIL

A hybrid of water mint and spearmint, peppermint contains the active ingredients menthone and menthol and is considered a mild stimulant. One of the world's oldest medicinal herbs, peppermint was used by the ancient Egyptians as well as in China, Japan, and Europe. One of the most versatile essential oils on the market, its properties range from repelling mosquitoes[19] to alleviating migraines and mitigating the side effects of cancer treatments. Peppermint is also a potent antioxidant.[20]

In terms of weight management, inhaling peppermint can reduce or eliminate food cravings and help you feel full faster, thus reducing caloric intake. It is particularly effective at blocking PMS cravings for chocolate and other sweets.[21] Peppermint is also a natural—and almost instantaneous—energizer, providing the get-up-and-go necessary to burn off calories without the sugar and toxins in energy drinks. It is a key ingredient in Mama Z's Fat-Burning Roll-On (page 275).

Try for Yourself: Make a hunger-curbing, energy-boosting aromatherapy inhaler by simply adding twenty drops of peppermint oil to the cotton swab that comes with your inhaler, insert it into the tube, and secure it with the lid for on-the-go benefit. Between meals, simply open the inhaler and take a few deep breaths of the vapor to keep you energized and help tame cravings for unhealthy foods.

4. CINNAMON ESSENTIAL OIL

Traditionally extracted from the *Cinnamomum zeylanicum* tree, cinnamon oil comes from either the inner bark or the leaves. (The source should be indicated on the bottle.) The leaf typically contains more eugenol, which is used to relieve pain and inflammation and fight bacteria. The bark is composed more of cinnamaldehyde and camphor, both potent as antioxidants and antidiabetics, meaning they help lower fasting blood-sugar levels.[22] The spice cinnamon has similar properties.[23]

Cinnamaldehyde has been shown to reduce blood glucose, a known cause of obesity and weight gain.[24] Another compound, cinnamic acid, improves glucose tolerance and has the potential to stimulate insulin production.[25] Both offer promise as remedies for type 2 diabetes, which is associated with excess weight.

Try for Yourself: Add a drop of cinnamon essential oil to our Fat-Burning Matcha Latte (page 215). The cinnamon has the added benefit of balancing your blood sugar level, which will help to minimize cravings.

The Power of Teamwork

One of the most intriguing things about essential oils is their ability to *synergize*—the phenomenon in which combinations of oils create even more potent healing properties than they possess individually. This is a fundamental concept behind creating blends. In 2005, George-town University Medical Center researchers took note of the benefits of synergy when they studied using essential oils to lower elevated blood sugar. Instead of isolating a single oil for their research, they experimented with blends of multiple oils that have been suggested as beneficial for diabetes.[26] We like this animal study for a couple reasons: it highlights the synergistic power of blending, and it provides the surprising benefits of using essential oils the right way.

The following three blends were tested:

1. E1: Oregano, cinnamon, fenugreek, cumin, and fennel
2. E2: Oregano, cinnamon, fenugreek, cumin, myrtle, allspice, and ginger
3. E3: Oregano, cinnamon, fenugreek, cumin, and myrtle

Each blend was mixed with pumpkinseed oil (an unusual carrier oil) and extra-virgin olive oil. A control group of rats received only water. The other three groups were given two or three drops orally of these essential oil blends in the carrier oil. (Smaller animals received two drops and larger animals received three drops.) All three blends demonstrated significantly improved insulin sensitivity, systolic blood pressure, and reduced weight, with the E3 group producing the most dramatic results.[27]

Try for Yourself: Make our Blood Sugar–Balancing Capsules (page 279) and take one capsule twice daily for two weeks. Consider trying the oils from the E3 blend above first, and work with your health-care provider to monitor your results.

Beyond the Basic Four

Once you familiarize yourself with the top four weight-management essential oils, you may want to branch out and try other scents, such as these other citrus oils: orange, lemon, tangerine, tangelo, clementine, mandarin orange, and neroli. Orange oil is an effective mood booster[28] and can help you avoid resorting to food for a lift. Bergamot, the oil that gives Earl Grey tea its distinctive scent and flavor, has been the subject of considerable research. Among its many benefits are enhanced weight loss,[29] stress relief,[30] and anxiety reduction.[31]

THE JURY IS STILL OUT ON LAVENDER OIL

In contrast to the four oils we have just discussed in depth, lavender has been shown to *stimulate* appetite, *slow* thermogenesis, *decrease* lipolysis, and *increase* body weight in rats.[32] However, in her book *Clinical Aromatherapy*, Jane Buckle, PhD, RN, reports on a 2005 study her students conducted that suggests the opposite.[33]

Of the thirty volunteers in this study, ten were asked to inhale lavender oil before meals and when food cravings occurred; another ten were asked to inhale mandarin orange oil; and the remaining ten (the control group) were asked to inhale grapeseed oil, which has no scent. The volunteers were asked to do this for six weeks while maintaining their eating habits. At the conclusion of the trial, the control group had lost on average 1.2 pounds, the mandarin orange group lost on average 2.4 pounds, and the lavender group lost 5.3 pounds.

At a quick glance, it would be easy to conclude that humans respond to lavender differently than animals do, which would explain why these two studies report conflicting results. However, that seems like an oversimplification. We all have different biochemical makeups, and you need to find what works for you.

If you're a stress-eater, then lavender could very well help you lose weight by minimizing anxiety and your tendency to use food to cope. Keep an inhaler on hand (in your purse, at your office, in your car) for quick on-the-go support and take some deep, relaxing breaths to help curb your tendency to grab an unhealthy snack when you're stressed.

If you find that lavender is so relaxing that it puts you in that calm and collected "parasympathetic mode" in which your body craves more food (especially snacks), steer clear of it until late in the evening, when you want your body and mind to start to cool down so you can get a good night's rest.

Root Cause Resolution

To really win the battle of the bulge, you need to get to the root causes. Eating healthful food full of bioactive compounds isn't going to do the trick if you are self-medicating by bingeing on those good foods and couch surfing. Following are some of the most common risk factors for weight gain. We'll show you how easy it is to use essential oils to address a number of these root causes, among them a sedentary lifestyle, elevated blood sugar, stress, chronic inflammation, anxiety, and gut disturbances.

GET MOVIN'!

A sedentary lifestyle is a major risk factor for being overweight. One common reason people don't like to exercise is because they don't know what they are doing and aren't getting the results they are hoping for. Don't worry, we've got you covered! Turn to Part 3 for a complete exercise plan that we use to keep in shape and stay fit!

Another excuse people use not to exercise is that they are too tired or unmotivated. We have already discussed how peppermint oil can give you the impetus to hop off the couch and get moving, so this is a good place to start! Peppermint oil can also instantly improve performance, endurance, and respiration rate.[34,35] In addition, it helps expand lung capacity, which means you can take in more oxygen, enabling your body to burn fat more efficiently.

If you are new to exercise, your initial enthusiasm can lead to overexertion and resultant muscle aches and pains. Topical applications of both peppermint and lavender oil are proven pain relievers.[36,37]

Try for Yourself: Make a muscle rub ointment by mixing six drops each of lavender and peppermint oils, and three drops each of copaiba and wintergreen oils, in a small glass container with 1 ounce of jojoba oil. Then rub it into sore muscles after you exercise for instant relief.

Both high and low blood sugar have been associated with weight gain, which is why you want to focus on *balancing* your body's physiology with essential oils and bioactive-rich foods.

Periods of low blood sugar foster cravings for sugary foods, making it a major cause of obesity, but the use of certain oils can help minimize those swings. One prominent study out of Georgetown University Medical Center took note of the benefits of synergy when they studied essential oils to help moderate type 2 diabetes. Instead of isolating a single oil for their research, they experimented with blends of such oils as cinnamon bark, cumin, fenugreek, and oregano and determined that various blends of these oils demonstrated great success in their ability to lower circulating blood-glucose levels and enhance insulin sensitivity.[38]

Other oils known for their blood sugar–balancing prowess include clove,[39] lavender, melissa[40] (lemon balm), and lemongrass. We have found that our Blood Sugar–Balancing blends (page 278) are key to keeping excess weight down if you're battling blood sugar concerns.

There is another way that essential oils can help with type 2 diabetes, particularly for people who also need to lose weight. Unhealthy weight gain and obesity are well-known risk factors for type 2 diabetes and the development of cardiovascular disease. As you would expect, obesity is associated with lipid accumulation in adipose (fat) cells. However, problems become severe when lipids accumulate in non-adipose tissues such as skeletal muscle and liver cells.

Research tells us that melissa is one of the most effective essential oils at inhibiting lipid accumulation into non-adipose tissue. Other honorable mentions include bergamot, black pepper,[41] cypress, geranium, lavender, niaouli, peppermint, and ravensara oils.[42]

Try for Yourself: Our recipe for Blood Sugar–Balancing Body Oil (page 279) will help moderate those swings, which can prompt cravings.

ESSENTIAL OILS FOR BALANCING BLOOD SUGAR

The key to using essential oils for type 2 diabetes and chronic blood sugar issues is to switch up your protocols regularly. As a rule of thumb, you'll want to change the oils or blends that you are using every three to four weeks. The oils below are known for their blood sugar-balancing efficacy, and you can start by blending two or three together to apply on your abdomen twice a day.

In Part 3, you will find recipes and blends that we have found to be helpful.

1. Bergamot
2. Black pepper
3. Cinnamon bark
4. Cumin
5. Cypress
6. Fenugreek
7. Geranium
8. Lavender
9. Lemongrass
10. Melissa (lemon balm)
11. Niaouli
12. Oregano
13. Peppermint
14. Ravensara

MANAGE STRESS AND ANXIETY

Stress doesn't just trigger cravings for unhealthy foods; it is also a huge factor in overall poor health. Among the essential oils that help you de-stress is lavender, which you already know as a sleep aid. You also now understand that inadequate shut-eye can prompt weight gain.

Anxiety can also lead to overeating or eating unhealthy foods. Thanks to its well-known antianxiety benefits, bergamot is often dubbed "liquid Xanax."[43] There are several other oils that can also help with anxiety. A 2015 systematic review of the review suggest that the following are the most potent:[44]

- Angelica
- Basil
- Bergamot
- Geranium
- Labdanum
- Lavender
- Lemon-scented ironbark
- May chang
- Orange
- Palmarosa
- Patchouli
- Petitgrain
- Sweet marjoram
- Sweet orange
- Valerian

Other studies also credit clary sage, lemon, Roman chamomile, rose, rose-scented geranium, sandalwood, and ylang-ylang with anti-anxiety effects.[45,46] Essential oils that make you feel calm and collected will help you manage anxiety. In turn, you will feel less inclined to stress-eat by snacking on unhealthy foods and generally running to food as a coping mechanism when anxiety settles in.

Try for Yourself: Add two drops each of valerian, geranium, and patchouli to a diffuser to reduce stress and anxiety.

TAME INFLAMMATION

Inflammation is your body's normal response to an injury or other attack; however *chronic inflammation* causes fat cells to transmit chemical messengers that can block other messengers, namely insulin and leptin. When the insulin messenger doesn't get through to your brain, you can't process insulin properly, leading to fat storage. And when leptin is blocked, your brain's signals that you are full and should stop eating are rendered inoperative. There are dozens of essential oils that are known to tame inflammation, and the first step is to create an inflammation blend that suits your desires. Here are some of the main anti-inflammatory components to look out for[47]:

- 1,8-cineole—found in eucalyptus *(Eucalyptus globulus* and *E. radiata)*, niaouli, cajeput, cardamom, rosemary, and sage
- Anethole—found in anise, cedarwood, and fennel
- Borneol—found in lavender, rosemary, lavandin, spike lavender, and sage
- Eugenol—found in clove, black pepper, and basil

In addition to the chemical components above, the following essential oils have been shown to have very promising anti-inflammatory properties according to research studies:[48]

- Caraway[49]
- Clove[50]
- Eucalyptus[51]
- Ginger[52]
- Lavender[53]
- Marjoram[54]
- Oregano[55]
- Peppermint[56]
- Roman chamomile[57]
- Tea tree[58]
- Thyme[59]
- Turmeric[60]

When using these anti-inflammatory oils, you'll more than likely discover that certain blends will work better for you than others.

Try for Yourself: Check out pages 283–285 for information about these anti-inflammatory preparations: anti-inflammation blend, inhaler, roll-on, and capsules.

Not only does eating the standard American diet (SAD) increase the likelihood of being overweight, but those foods and beverages, along with stress, inactivity, and other factors inherent in our contemporary lifestyle, can damage your gut. In turn, such damage can make it difficult to achieve and maintain a healthy weight. However, you will find that the following essential oils are of specific help on your path to healing.

- *Peppermint.* Traditionally known as an excellent digestive remedy, peppermint essential oil has long been indicated for irritable bowel syndrome (IBS) via enteric-coated capsules.[61] Coriander and lemon balm oils have also shown to be effective.[62]
- *Thyme.* An antimicrobial by day, a gut healer by night, thyme is a superhero essential oil. Both thymol (in thyme) and geraniol (in rose oil) are effective in suppressing pathogens in the small intestine, without harming "good" gut bacteria.[63]
- *Lavender.* Once again, this essential oil comes to the fore with its dual ability to improve gut health as well as relieve the anxiety that can contribute to gut problems.
- *Cumin.* This essential oil has been shown to reduce pain, bloating, and elimination problems, among other benefits.[64]

These four may be the superstars of the digestive oils, but others deserve some of the limelight. Ginger is a standout for nausea and initial digestive complaints. As mentioned earlier, citrus oils are gentle and effective for both digestion and such peripheral issues as anxiety and microbial concerns. If you're serious about rebuilding your gut, essential oils should be a key tool in your wellness kit.

Purity Is Key

It should go without saying that only pure essential oils can help you reach your health goals, including achieving a healthy weight. Not only is your body incapable of properly metabolizing synthetic oils, but also improper use may produce such adverse reactions as inflammation or an allergy, or even compromise your immune system.

Moreover, even a pure essential oil may not produce the desired effect if there are chemicals in it that don't interact well with the chemicals in your body. Aromatherapy is a very individual practice, and bio-individuality means that what works for one person doesn't necessarily do so for another.

Here's how to choose a reputable oil brand:

1. *Get a referral.* Ask someone you trust and respect which are their favorite brands. Marketing plays a major role in this industry, so you need to separate the hype from the reality. If someone is selling a specific brand of essential oils, she is almost certainly biased. On the other hand, if you find you keep hearing certain brands recommended by different (and unrelated) people, one or more may well be worth sampling.

2. *Research sourcing and quality control policies.* Once you find a company that interests you, research the sources of its raw materials and what quality-control measures are used. Larger companies may provide such information on their website, but you may need to speak to an informed person at a smaller company or request a report via e-mail. If your inquiries are ignored or given short shrift, you would be wise to look for a more responsive company.

3. *Request a batch report.* A gas chromatography/mass spectrometry (GC/MS) report is a graph that can reveal adulteration and displays the chemical makeup of a specific oil, which can alert you to synthetic ingredients. Ask the company for a report on several of the oils that you're interested in to assist in determining their potential health benefits as well as any safety issues.

4. *Sample some.* Purchase at least two brands to see if you like them. Lime, grapefruit, cinnamon, and peppermint essential oils are among the less expensive oils. Test them by observing how your body responds when you inhale, feel, and taste

the oil. If, for example, a bottle of peppermint oil gives you a headache right off the bat, it simply means that your body isn't responding well to a chemical in a species of the herb from a certain locale or that was harvested at a certain time of year. These are just some of the factors that can impact your response. You might well be fine with the grapefruit oil of the same brand. Try another brand of peppermint until you find a compatible one.

Your body responds to any essential oil via six senses: taste, touch, smell, sight, hearing, and intuition, in what is called an organoleptic evaluation. You should check out your body's responses every time you get a new oil to ensure that the chemicals sync with your chemistry.

Now that you've had a taste for—or should we say a scent for—essential oils, you'll probably want to learn more about how to use them for even a wider variety of risk factors for weight gain, as well as to address other health concerns. If so, pick up Dr. Z's first book, *The Healing Power of Essential Oils*.

In the next chapter, we'll delve into the Essential Lifestyle, the program you will be following for the rest of your healthy and fit life.

CHAPTER 7

FOREVER TRANSFORM YOUR LIFE AND HEALTH WITH THE ESSENTIAL LIFESTYLE

"We first make our habits, and then our habits make us."
—JOHN DRYDEN

Welcome to the second phase—although we prefer to call it the rest of your life!—of the Essential Oils Diet. Congratulations! Whether or not you have lost all the weight you hoped to shed in the Fast Track, you have begun the process of healing your body and learning new, healthy habits.

Now it is time to segue to the Essential Lifestyle, although if you want to shed some more pounds and feel you can continue to comply with the relative rigor of the Fast Track, you can certainly hang out there a bit longer. It's up to you. Again, you get to personalize your own program.

In this chapter you'll discover how to catapult off the success that you have already gained on the Fast Track, and we'll show you how to tweak things to your liking so you can stay in this "phase" for the rest of your life! These easy-to-follow tips and practical strategies will all but ensure that you will enjoy a healthy weight for many years to come, regardless of whether you're pregnant, eating out, traveling, going to school, or simply when life happens.

Phase Two of Your Transformation: Honing New Habits

When you decide to transition from the Fast Track to the Lifestyle, you'll still want to follow the Eight Essential Habits that you learned beginning on page 95. Now is the time to fine-tune the other new habits you have been practicing. You'll continue to focus on eating healthy, nutritious foods that are devoid of toxins, which will enable your body to fall into a natural rhythm and reach its natural healthy weight.

Remember, you hold in your hands the power to make a difference. The biggest thing that we have learned from this whole process is that we have to be willing to do things that most people won't do to get the results that most people won't get:

- There are no built-in cheat days as there are with many diets. If you do briefly fall off the program, get right back in the saddle. And don't wallow in guilt, which could make you lose your resolve to stay the course. This is a marathon, not a sprint, okay?
- Continue to eat until you're pleasantly full, but not stuffed. No more gorging, no more Clean Plate Club.
- If you have been fasting intermittently, continue to make it a way of life. If you did not begin fasting in the Essential Fast Track, start with juice fasting and work your way up to a day of consuming only water once a week or once a month.
- After thirty days on the Fast Track, you should be having regular bowel movements. Think of colon cleansing like changing the oil on your car. Get a colonic or do an enema once or twice a year or when you know something is "off." A good sign that you need to clean your colon is chronic fatigue, regular pain, brain fog, or such digestive concerns as constipation, diarrhea, and bloating. (See Cleanse Your Colon: Personalize Your Program on page 111.)
- Essential oils should be part of your daily routine by now. Take a deep dive into their therapeutic, fat-burning power and

check out the recipes in Part 3 for healing remedies that you can make.

- Continue getting sun or supplementing with a vitamin D supplement. Consider buying a supplement paired with vitamin K_2, as research suggests they work synergistically to promote heart and bone health.[1] We take one that combines 2,500 IU of vitamin D_3 plus 100 mcg of vitamin K_2 during the winter months when we don't get a lot of sun exposure.
- Regular movement and exercise should be a way of life. Keep up your walking, increasing the distance and pace if possible. Likewise, try out new exercises and/or increase the number of sets and reps you have been doing. If you haven't already done so, consider enrolling in a group exercise class. Or better yet, start to implement Mama Z's exercise program in Part 3 and kick it up a notch!
- Take your healthy sleeping habits to the next level and start to tackle advanced strategies such as reducing EMFs (electromagnetic frequencies) and other known sleep disruptors from your life. We cover these tips and more in chapter 8.

Focus on eating healthy, nutritious foods, and your body will naturally fall into a rhythm and reach its optimal weight. Learn how to read labels scrupulously. (See Buyer Beware: Learn to Read Labels on page 149.) And free yourself from an obsession with the scale. Weigh yourself once a month, if at all. Let the way your clothes fit be your guide.

As you may recall from chapter 1, it takes an average of sixty-six days for a habit to become completely ingrained, so be patient with yourself—especially if you slip! If you do fall back into old habits, don't beat yourself up: "For the righteous falls seven times and rises again" *(Proverbs 24:16)*! Like children learning to walk, we need to understand that "falling" is part of the process.

We are all "under construction," so to speak, so always keep in mind that the Essential Lifestyle is a marathon, not a sprint. "The path of the righteous is like the morning sun, shining ever brighter till the full light of day" *(Proverbs 4:18)*. Think of your time on earth as beginning like a "sunrise" and ending as a life-giving "high noon." Embrace the journey, knowing that you will be a beacon of light for your loved ones if you stay true to the course.

Embed these two proverbs in your heart as a source of strength and encouragement if and when you're tempted to beat yourself up or quit when you trip and fall.

To help you get started on the Essential Lifestyle, we have compiled an Essential Lifestyle Success Package—which includes a starter checklist, a shopping guide, and a meal plan— that you can download by visiting EssentialOilsDiet.com.

What's on and off the Menu?

Now that "boot camp" is over, you will be able to eat a wider array of food, which is not to say that you can go back to your old way of eating. Fake, processed, and chemical-filled "foods" continue to have no place in your new lifestyle.

Raw dairy products are fine, and you can start to enjoy more grains and the occasional sweet treat. You many have enjoyed some of the sweet treats acceptable in the Fast Track. Mama Z has cooked up some more naturally sweetened treats that will please your sweet tooth in the Essential Lifestyle. We'll get into greater detail on the following pages. Remember the big picture: The real objective is to form permanent habits that lead you down the path to transformation.

The key here is not to restrict yourself so you feel like you're on a diet. The reason we don't eat bad foods is because we understand that they are bad for us and we want to consume things that promote vitality and life. Now let's take a closer look:

- *Alcohol.* Even with the occasional glass of wine at meals, there is no value in drinking alcohol, and it doesn't fit in the

Essential Lifestyle. There are more health risks associated with liquor than there are apparent benefits. Functional medicine practitioners consider alcohol to be an *antinutrient*. Among the many reasons alcohol is not your friend is that it can create oxidative stress that contributes to bone loss[2] and can cause cancer.[3] Plus nothing else will give you a beer belly like . . . well, beer.

- *Breads and grains.* Now that you're past the Fast Track, don't slip back into the habit of making bread and other wheat foods a major component of your diet. Stick with truly gluten-free versions of pizza, sandwiches, or pancakes. Our recipes and pantry staples include some good commercial gluten-free products without added sugars and additives. If it is difficult to find them locally, order them online at Thrive Market (see page 91). Unless you are traveling to Europe, steer clear of all wheat products. (Remember, the weed-killer glyphosate used on conventionally grown American wheat is banned in most European countries. Glyphosate destroys gut flora, causing inflammation, and may well be the cause of the ailments typically attributed to wheat itself.) Opt for organic (ideally sprouted) whole, ancient grains such as oatmeal, quinoa, millet, brown rice, spelt, amaranth, sorghum, and teff. Of course, moderation is key, and always stick with organic versions. Abusing any grains will cause the pounds to jump back on in a jiffy!

MAMA Z TIP

Nothing beats a sandwich for portability, but finding bread that's tasty and contains only acceptable ingredients is a challenge. I make my own whole-grain, gluten-free bread, but Sami's Bakery is a commercial option. At Target, we found Franz gluten-free breads, which come in three varieties: Cinnamon Raisin, Great Seed, and 7-Grain. Neither Sami's nor Franz's gluten-free breads contain sugar, as most others do (making them a no-no). If you are not gluten-intolerant, *you can also enjoy Ezekiel bread, which is organic and made with sprouted and fermented grains, in moderation, of course. Any bread can pack on the pounds if you overdo it.*

- *Dairy.* Primarily due to the way dairy cows are raised, we don't see much room for conventional dairy products in the Essential Lifestyle. The occasional piece of raw cheese is one thing, but drinking a gallon of cow's milk every week is quite another. For starters, pasteurized, hormone-fed, antibiotic-enriched milk products aren't safe for human consumption. Avoid them at all costs. The best options on the market for dairy lovers are organic, grass-fed, raw dairy products such as cheese, kefir, and yogurt. If you can't get your hands on raw milk products, be sure to buy only organic, grass-fed dairy. We have also found that most people can tolerate sheep and goat products much better than cow products. So feel free to enjoy goat cheese or Manchego with your tapas!
- *Meat.* The occasional poultry, lamb, or beef dish isn't going to hurt you, but don't make a habit of eating them. Again, the way most food animals are raised involves GMO grains and antibiotics at the very least. Seriously, try to limit your animal protein and fats and enjoy them as treats the way our Bible ancestors did for feast days, holidays, and special occasions.
- *Sweets.* In Part 3, you'll find a number of delectable, naturally sweetened treats straight from our kitchen. If you don't have the time or inclination to make your own, your local health food store will most likely offer goodies naturally sweetened with dates, honey, stevia, maple syrup, or coconut sugar.

As you did in the first phase, you'll want to come up with your own daily meal plans. On page 141 is a template to scan and print out. We suggest you post each day's meal plan on your refrigerator door. A sample Essential Lifestyle meal plan follows, to show how to use the recipes Mama Z has created to construct your own meal plans. You can also use the template that follows for your Essential Lifestyle weekly meal plans.

7-DAY ESSENTIAL LIFESTYLE MEAL PLAN

	Breakfast	Lunch	Dinner	Snack/Dessert
Monday				
Tuesday				
Wednesday				
Thursday				
Friday				
Saturday				
Sunday				

7-DAY ESSENTIAL LIFESTYLE MEAL PLAN

	Breakfast	Lunch	Dinner	Snack/Dessert
Monday	**Mama Z's Bioactive Breakfast Shake** (page 222)	**Quick Tuna or Salmon Salad** (page 226)	**Mama Z's Spaghetti with Meat Sauce*** (page 250) with gluten-free spaghetti and a side garden salad	**Lemon Dip with Essential Oils*** (page 238) with gluten-free crackers
Tuesday	**Greens and Herb Omelet** (page 222)	**Avocado Egg Salad** (page 226)	**South of the Border Casserole** (page 252) with fresh-cut veggies for dipping	**Fill in the Gap Nuts** (page 244)
Wednesday	**Berry Green Delight Smoothie** (page 224)	**Greens and Herb Omelet** (page 222)	Poached or grilled wild-caught salmon, brown basmati rice, and a side garden salad	**Mama Z's Hummus** (page 242) with fresh-cut veggies for dipping
Thursday	**Cacao Energy Bowl** (page 224)	**South of the Border Casserole** (page 252) with gluten-free taco chips	**Slow-Cooker Lasagna** (page 248) with gluten-free pasta and a side garden salad	**Superfood Peppermint Patties** (page 264)
Friday	Scrambled eggs with sliced tomato and avocado	**Super Greens Summer Salad** (page 228)	**Deluxe Fish Salad** (page 246)	**Easy Lemon Pie with Essential Oils*** (page 271)
Saturday	**Spicy Autumn Breakfast Bake*** (page 225)	**Super Greens Summer Salad** (page 228)	Olive, tomato, bell pepper, and nondairy mozzarella shreds on a cauliflower pizza crust	**Fill in the Gap Nuts** (page 244)
Sunday	**Heart-Healthy Blueberry Pancakes** (page 218)	**Deluxe Fish Salad** (page 246)	**Stuffed Portobello Mushroom Salad** (page 241)	**Dr. Z's Chocolate-Avocado Puddin'** (page 267)

TIME-SAVING MEAL-PREP TIPS

Mama Z here. Realistically, a busy family with working parents probably isn't going to make a new lunch and dinner each day. But preparing healthy food shouldn't be a problem if you follow the five *P*s: Proper Planning Prevents Poor Performance. Here's how to make the most of your precious time:

- *Develop an assembly-line approach.* Prepare two meals at once, eat one, and freeze the other. With a family of six, I often actually triple or quadruple meals. (Or if you are cooking for yourself or a small family, reheating a hot dish or reaching into the fridge for another serving a day or two later is a great time-saver, reflected in the meal plan on the previous page.) I like to devote a day a month or half a day each week to ready a bunch of dishes.

- *Involve your kids.* Even if they're too young to be trusted with a knife, they can measure ingredients or peel carrots. Yes, they will likely make a mess, but they'll have fun and begin to learn the importance of good food.

- *Perform some quick change artistry.* Reintroduce the side salad you had for dinner on Monday night as lunch on Tuesday with the addition of a couple of hard-boiled eggs, dairy-free cheese, or lentils. (Just don't dress the side salad before serving.) Or make Avocado Egg Salad (page 226) for lunch and have it as a snack on nut crackers the next day.

- *Plan on leftovers.* Reheat them a day or two later or add to a second dish. For example, my spaghetti sauce (see page 249) turns up again in lasagna (see page 247). Chop up leftover raw veggies to top a salad. Add leftover berries and chopped fruit to yogurt cups.

- *Think big by batch prepping.* Make a large pot of soup over the weekend, individually portion it for the next couple of days, then freeze the rest. Or keep it in the fridge and add any leftover veggies, rice, or pasta to the pot so you have a slightly different soup the next day, and maybe the day after.

- *Triple-wash enough salad greens* for several days and store them in separate ziplock bags for each day. Add a piece of paper towel to absorb excess moisture. You'll be able to put together a salad in a jiffy.
- *Let someone else do the work.* When I'm serving a salad to a crowd, I'll often rely on bagged organic spinach, kale, or power greens—as well as grated carrots and cabbage.
- *Serve breakfast for dinner.* Crustless quiche or savory almond-flour pancakes or waffles with chopped leftover cooked veggies are good any time of day.
- *Rely on healthy time-saving shortcuts* such as prepared cauliflower pizza crusts or dough mixes (Simple Mills pizza dough mix is made with almond flour). I'll top the pizza with tomato sauce and leftover veggies, olives, and nondairy cheese. Tetra Pak organic vegetable broth is another time-saver. Just combine it with leftovers from dinner the night before and you'll have a hearty soup in minutes.
- *Finally, invest in a separate freezer.* You'll need it to store extra meals as well as save money by buying certain items in bulk.

GOODBYE TO BAD EATING HABITS

As you shed some of your old food habits, you'll simultaneously be developing new ones on the path to transformation. Here are a few you may not have thought of:

- *Pray before your meals.* Giving thanks causes you to slow down and stop (for at least a minute or two) before you dive in and devour your food. By putting yourself in a more relaxed state, you'll enjoy your food more and digest it better.

- *Eat slowly and mindfully.* Create an opportunity to savor the tastes and textures of food. The satisfaction provided helps curb overeating because it gives your tummy more time to signal the sensation of fullness to your brain. Eating too fast is an invitation to eat too much.
- *Do one thing at a time.* Eating while watching TV, texting, using your computer, or any activity that takes your mind off enjoying your meal and paying attention to how much you are eating increases the likelihood of overeating.
- *No more after-dinner snacks.* Your gut needs a much-needed respite from the job of digestion. Plus, you may be inclined to eat sweets and other problematic foods late at night.
- *Stop the snacking habit altogether.* If you are eating nutritious meals, there should be no need to snack. It is more likely a crutch because you're bored or tired. You will be more aware of the flavors in your foods if you eat only at meal times, making them all the more enjoyable. On the other hand, if a snack will keep you on the straight and narrow, have at it. Just make sure it is a healthy one.
- *Use a salad plate.* A large dinner plate may tempt you to completely fill it up.
- *Keep treats out of sight.* That way you won't be enticed to eat things that you shouldn't. Yes, this includes healthy, naturally sweetened treats. Too much of a good thing is still too much, right?
- *Drink a glass of our essential oils sparkling water* (see page 219). When midday hunger pangs hit, it can help satisfy your tummy's need to feel full. This will also help you stay hydrated, so it's a win-win!

PROTEIN BARS—IN THEIR PROPER PLACE

Bars can come in handy when traveling. We look for those without soy, wheat, corn, dairy, or sugar, which considerably narrows the field. Four brands fit the bill:

- **Pegan Protein** bars derive their 20 grams of protein from pumpkin seeds and are sweetened with monk fruit. Ingredients are 98 percent organic, with no added sugar, sugar alcohols, corn, or dairy.
- **Living Fuel CocoChia** bars are made with organic ingredients and are free of GMOs, pesticides, and herbicides. The main ingredients are coconut, chia seeds, and almond butter, and the bars are sweetened with sugar alcohols and agave syrup.
- **Lärabars** contain no gluten, soy, or dairy, and are non-GMO. Some do contain sugar; others may contain milk in chocolate chips, so read each ingredient list before choosing a flavor. The Lemon bar is sweetened only with dates, and the Cherry Pie contains just dates, unsweetened cherries, and almonds. However, the Peanut Butter Chocolate Chip may have milk in the chips.
- **Julian Bakery** Paleo Thin Protein bars are made with egg-white protein and sweetened with monk fruit.

Haven't Lost (Much) Weight?

Have you lost inches in your waist, hips, chest, arms, and thighs? If you are exercising regularly you may not have lost as much weight as you had hoped, but the inches are actually just as important. If you have built up more muscle, it could offset the loss of some fat pounds, but you would still be ahead of the game.

If you still want to lose more weight, do you plan to stay in Fast Track for a little longer? Or are you willing to see the progress of your weight loss slow somewhat as you add back some of the foods we advised you to avoid for the first thirty days? As long as you eat until you are 80 percent full, you will likely continue to lose weight. You may plateau for a week or so before weight loss resumes, or it could mean you have reached the weight your body wants to be.

Assuming you followed the Essential Fast Track and the obvious reasons of overeating, being sedentary, or having a family history of being overweight do not apply, ask yourself these questions:

- *Are xenoestrogens, aka endocrine disruptors, at fault?* Hormone imbalance and environmental toxins are intricately intertwined, which is one reason that diabetes and obesity have been linked with toxic overload. Groundbreaking research by the American Diabetes Association has found low levels of six persistent organic pollutants (POPs) in the blood of more than 80 percent of adult volunteers.[4,5] One POP called oxychlordane is a pesticide used on citrus fruits and corn, as well as lawns and gardens. All six POPs had a strong association with diabetes and put the volunteers at risk for a higher BMI (body mass index) and waist circumference. The researchers estimated that 90 percent of these POPs come from the meat of conventionally raised animals fed GMO grain and soy sprayed with these pesticides. If you have been eating conventional meat products regularly, replace them with the occasional certified organic, grass-fed beef dish, and eat less meat overall. Likely, you'll see your weight loss back on track.

- *Is poor digestion a factor?* In order to shed—and keep off—excess pounds, your digestive system must be in tiptop condition, enabling your body to absorb nutrients and remove waste. "Gastrointestinal and digestive issues can definitely have a large effect on the way we eat and how our bodies absorb and digest foods, causing us to gain or lose weight," says Kenneth Brown, MD, a board-certified gastroenterologist. "Most digestive problems tend to cause weight loss from poor absorption of food, but there are a few situations in which our intestinal health can contribute to weight gain."[6] The main culprits are acid reflux or gastroesophageal reflux disease (GERD), ulcers, constipation, bacterial overgrowth, irritable bowel syndrome, ulcerative colitis, Crohn's disease, and food intolerance. Consider visiting a functional medicine doctor for an evaluation and advice on a holistic treatment plan to address the root cause of excess weight gain.

- *Are you taking antibiotics or other drugs that can interfere with weight loss?* We've known for years that antibiotic exposure promotes fat gain in animals.[7] More recently, researchers have uncovered that antibiotic use in the first six months of life contributes to increased weight well into childhood and possibly through adulthood.[8,9] Discuss any medications you are on with your health-care provider, and see if you can switch to another drug or reduce your dosage. Another reason not to eat meat from conventionally raised animals is that a few weeks before being slaughtered, they are fed antibiotics to encourage weight gain.

- *Are you experiencing systemic inflammation?* If you find yourself tired all of the time; battling brain fog, digestive complaints, and skin issues such as psoriasis and eczema; and always struggling with seasonal allergies, chances are that you are suffering from chronic, systemic inflammation. Inflammation is also a factor in uncontrolled weight gain, increased abdominal fat, and metabolic syndrome.[10,11] Research has already proven beyond a shadow of a doubt that an inflammatory diet greatly contributes to weight gain. Conversely, following our anti-inflammatory dietary guidelines laid out in the Essential Oils Diet can help soothe your system and make it easier to sustain weight loss. To speed up the process and reduce stress, pray, meditate, and combat inflammation by using essential oils. We describe the anti-inflammatory recipes you'll want to use in Part 3.

BUYER BEWARE: LEARN TO READ LABELS

Most manufacturers provide the least amount of information required to comply with government regulations. Chemical companies and major food manufacturers have fought hard to avoid or minimize language that could alert an increasingly aware public to the presence of certain ingredients or processes. Moreover, the information on labels required by law is often of little use to the average person. To read between the lines, this is what you should look for:

- *GMO ingredients.* Look for the words *non-GMO* and assume all other products may contain genetically modified organisms. Produce that is GMO is tagged with a five-digit number starting with an 8.
- *Natural.* There is no legal definition for this term, making it meaningless. Arsenic is natural, but you wouldn't want it in your food or household products!
- *Organic.* This term can be used even if only 95 percent or more of a product is organic. Products that are 100 percent organic are labeled as such. Fresh produce that is organic is tagged with a five-digit number that starts with a 5. Conventionally grown produce bears a four-digit number.
- *Grass fed.* This refers to meat or dairy products raised on grass and forage. ("Grass finished" means the animal was fed a conventional diet of grain and soy until shortly before being slaughtered, when its diet was changed.) However, a loophole in the law allows the use of the label even if the animal has spent some of its life in a pen or if a company was using such a label before the 2007 standard was created. Again, your best bet is to purchase meat from a local farmer whom you know practices what he preaches.
- *Free range.* According to the USDA, this terminology can be used only for chickens and other animals, not for eggs. In any case, it is meaningless, ensuring only that there is a door through which a chicken theoretically departs, potentially

spending no more than a few minutes a day outside—and then only if it could push its way past hundreds, if not thousands, of other hens. Nor does it ensure the chickens are raised organically. The Humane Farm Animal Care (HFAC) program is the only one that actually certifies poultry as "free range," ensuring that, weather permitting, birds spend at least six hours a day outside. (Their diet is also organic.) Pens must also allow each chicken at least 2 square feet of space.

- *Pasture raised.* The HFAC is also the only organization that offers this certification, requiring that each bird has at least 108 square feet and is outdoors year-round in rotating fields. In extremely inclement weather or to protect them from predators, chickens may be provided with shelter.

Eating Well When Eating Out

The remainder of this chapter is devoted to sharing simple, practical tips we have adopted over the years that will help empower you to deal with many of the situations that cause so many people to fall off the wagon. We will address going to restaurants, navigating the minefield of indulgent holiday dishes, and figuring out what to eat while traveling.

First up: going out to eat! To get the meal you want without ingredients you don't, speak up. Restaurants are a service industry; it is their job to serve you what you want—or at least inform you of what is possible. If the server seems unsure about the ingredients in a dish, ask if you can talk to the chef. Restaurants are as concerned with food allergies and food sensitivities as you are and will be more than glad to accommodate.

And do your homework. Check out a restaurant's website and call ahead to determine if the staff is amenable to handling a diner's requests and whether it proudly declares that it serves organic foods and wild-caught fish.

Chipotle Mexican Grill, Panera Bread, Jason's Deli, Seasons 52, and Ruby Tuesday are just a few of the many chain restaurants where you can get a healthy meal if you ask the right questions. All of them offer dishes designed for people with certain allergies. Ruby Tuesday's salad bar is truly fresh (see below) and has an excellent selection of organic greens and other vegetables. At Chipotle, everything is made to order. Most of the produce is locally sourced and organic (and therefore non-GMO), although the meat and poultry are not, so we only order the veggie bowl and opt for brown rice, black beans, fajita veggies, guacamole, non-GMO corn, lettuce, and either pico de gallo or salsa verde.

Our go-to meal when eating out at other restaurants is usually a big salad topped with wild-caught fish, steamed or grilled with sea salt, pepper, and a squeeze of lemon or lime. Steer clear of the salad dressings and stick with olive oil and balsamic vinegar. A baked sweet potato makes a great side dish, and load up on the side veggies. Dessert is a fresh fruit plate.

When a wedding, business luncheon, or another event is on your calendar, call the coordinator of the facility ahead of time to find out about special meal options such as fish, vegetarian, vegan, or gluten-free. If you are not a vegetarian or vegan, reserve the fish entree (grilled or steamed salmon preferably) and ask for a double portion of vegetables. When you arrive, remind the coordinator of your special meal and point out where you are sitting. We have always found the staff willing to accommodate our needs.

A smoothie can make a great breakfast, but be aware that most places routinely add sugar or syrup. Make it clear you want neither and request unsweetened almond or coconut milk. Be sure to include avocado and kale (and/or spinach) as well as your preferred fruits. If smoothies aren't an option, get a veggie omelet cooked in butter or olive oil and a side of breakfast potatoes with some fruit.

Here are some more eating-out tips:

- Check with your server or maître d' to ensure that the salad bar or salad greens are really fresh, meaning they have not been sprayed with sulfites to *appear* fresh after sitting around for days.

- If tilapia is on the menu, pass it up. Almost always a farmed fish, it is fed fish meal full of GMO grains and is often contaminated with heavy metals and multiple other toxins.
- When you need to find a good place to eat in an unfamiliar area, head for the local health food store. It may have a cafe, or the proprietor can recommend a nearby organic, vegan, or vegetarian restaurant.
- You never know what is in salad dressing. Instead, bring your own in a sealed container and ask for your salad "naked."
- Also carry a small bottle of liquid stevia to sweeten tea, smoothies, or fruit, as needed.

Eating Healthy While Traveling

The precept of Proper Planning Prevents Poor Performance comes into play again when we're on the road with four children. Once you come up with a procedure that works smoothly, you should be able to travel with minimal hassle.

- *Develop a standing packing list for food-related items.* Keep it on your computer so you don't have to reinvent the wheel each time you travel. Simply cross off any items you know will be at your destination.
- *Learn the lay of the land.* Well before you depart, inquire about which appliances are in the kitchen/kitchenette at the hotel or Airbnb. Is there a full-size fridge, or can an additional bar fridge be provided? What pots and pans are available? Is there a blender? If necessary, we bring our two-burner hot plate to a hotel.
- *Bring travel meals.* To save money and time and avoid chain restaurant food, make travel meals ahead and bring them in a cooler. A combo heater/cooler—it sits between the front seats and plugs into the console—keeps food warm on the road. It can also serve as an extra "oven" at your destination.

- *Bring healthy snacks.* Our cooler is usually filled with salad, fruit cups, yogurt cups, applesauce, cut-up veggies, shakes, and beverages. We also bring Mama Z's Fill in the Gap Nuts (page 244), crackers and cookies made with almond flour, grain-free tortilla chips, and fruit and veggie squeeze pouches.
- *To each his own.* Each child has his or her own insulated lunch box for lunch and dinner as well, if we have a long drive.
- *Make meals ahead.* Freeze individual portions and use them as extra freezer packs on the road. Defrost and eat after you arrive at your destination.
- *Make breakfast hassle-free.* Bring breakfast for the morning after you arrive. Our kids love organic puffed oat and rice cereals and grain-free organic granola. (For more ideas, see Mama Z's Kitchen Makeover on page 206.) Smoothies are one of our favorite breakfasts, or we make omelets ahead of time, place them in the cooler, and reheat as needed.
- *Bring specialty items.* Pack foods that could be difficult to find at your destination. Our "go bag" is filled with supplies that always travel with us, such as oil, vinegar, raw honey, stevia, matcha green tea, cacao, and maca powder. We also bring organic butter and healthy mustard, ketchup, and pickle relish in the cooler bag.
- *Be considerate.* If you are staying with friends or family, coordinate in advance about what you need to bring. Some people will welcome your supplying much of your own food; others could feel offended. Patiently explain the special food needs of your family, and they will most likely understand. Also discuss the logistics of using someone else's kitchen.
- *It never hurts to ask.* Hotels are increasingly aware of special dietary needs, and many chains are geared to family travel. For example, the kitchen staff at Embassy Suites will prepare eggs with our ingredients if we ask.

MAMA Z TIP

We don't eat at McDonald's, but on a family trip we'll stop for a bathroom break and let the kids use the PlayPlace. Or we'll all get out of the car and do push-ups at a rest stop.

Bon Voyage: Eating Healthy Abroad

Mama Z here. When we go overseas, I pack a food suitcase with staples such as organic nut butters and manuka honey so I can easily make sandwiches for the kids. I'll also bring stevia, nut snacks, raisins and other dried fruit, and even some Tetra Pak items such as almond or coconut milk. We tend to eat dinner at restaurants, but making our own breakfasts and lunches minimizes the chance that one of the kids will get sick.

Here's some other advice:

- If the hotel has a policy against bringing in outside food, explain that you or someone in your family has food allergies—don't use the word *sensitivities*! Usually their attitude is "We don't want to mess with this. We need to help them."

- Be clear when you make a hotel reservation that you will need extra refrigeration. Sometimes that means a real refrigerator, but if a minibar fridge is the only option, ask if you can have a second one. Once, when all we had was a minibar fridge, I simply took everything out and put our food in it. It was a challenge, but we managed.
- I also always bring my trusty travel electric kettle. Don't forget an adapter.
- After we drink a bottle of kombucha or Voss water, we recycle the bottles to hold nut milks or other liquids; the bottles take up less space than the original containers.
- Short term, an ice bucket can come in handy if refrigerator space is at a premium.
- At home I make my own produce wash, but abroad I bring Gowipe Fruit n Veggie Wipes. Or I'll put a drop or two of essential oil in with just a tiny bit of unscented dish detergent and warm water to clean fruit and veggies. Be sure to rinse them thoroughly.

MAMA Z TIP

When we are traveling, I always make sure to have some of the little vacuum-packed packets of tuna and salmon to top a salad or serve as a filling for sandwiches.

How to Handle Holidays

Mama Z here. Celebrating holidays is wonderful, but the types of food often associated with these events, to say nothing of the sheer quantity offered, can be challenging when you are following any weight-loss program or simply trying to maintain your weight. Here's how we navigate those tricky shoals.

- *Never upstage your host.* Ask well in advance what's on the menu and what you can bring. So if you know that it's a Butterball turkey pumped full of antibiotics and raised on GMO corn, offer to bring a dish such as gluten-free, dairy-free macaroni and cheese that can be regarded as a side dish. That way, you're not casting any aspersions on her turkey.

- *Don't overlap.* If someone else is making mashed potatoes, offer to bring an equivalent dish, such as my Spiced Butternut Squash Soufflé★ (page 231).
- *Offer options.* For example, if I'm hosting, I'll make my grandma's traditional macaroni and cheese, but I'll also do gluten- and dairy-free versions. Or I might do a version of lasagna with grass-fed ground beef and another with spinach.
- *Bread and dessert are always welcome.* Plus if you make it or select it, you won't regret it the next day. People are usually amazed at how great a loaf of fresh-baked gluten-free bread tastes!
- *Ditto for dips.* You can never go wrong with bringing a veggie tray and a couple of healthy dips like hummus and lemon dip. (See page 211 for some of my delectable dips.)

To watch Mama Z make her famous hummus dip and to get tips on how to make tasty variations of this traditional dish, visit EssentialOilsDiet.com.

Avoiding Holiday Temptation

Food and communal dining play a major role in celebrating holidays. It's wonderful to "break bread" with those near and dear, but that celebratory environment can also create challenges if you are in the process of changing your relationship with food. How do you stay in control when temptation beckons?

- *Set yourself up for success.* Most of the time, it's eating after you're already full that causes problems. If you know that

Aunt Harriet's chocolate chip cookies—or whatever is your stumbling block—will be there, bring your own healthier version. Have just one as a treat and then hand them around to others. Be sure to leave your cookies behind, although chances are they will have been devoured!

- *Balance eating with activity.* If you're consuming more sweet or starchy foods, also commit to spending more time at the gym or doing whatever you can to burn off some of that extra fuel. Join in a family game of touch football, or take some long brisk walks with your sister-in-law.

- *Fast before a feast.* Most people aren't tempted to overeat protein, but I do regularly hear "Bread is my downfall." Or pasta, or cookies, or sweets, which, of course, are all present at holiday gatherings. We recommend a ten- to fourteen-day "vacation" from high-carb foods or whatever trigger food is the culprit *before* the holidays, plus a few days of transition. Doing so will provide clarity on the effect such foods have on you, which can strengthen your resolve and help break your "addiction."

- *Follow a feast with a fast.* People often decide to fast *after* a holiday, which is fine, but don't use it as an excuse to gorge over the holiday. You always want to transition into a fast of any sort, which argues for moderation before you begin.

- *Fill up on water.* If you struggle with overeating or know the food isn't going to be that healthy, drink a big glass of water spiked with lemon essential oil before you head out for a holiday meal. Sip some more before you sit down to curb your appetite. On the other hand, as long as the food is healthy, eat until you feel comfortably full but not stuffed. (See No Need to Count Anything on page 70.)

Preparing for Weddings and Other Special Events

Mama Z here. Of course you want to be in optimal shape when you go to a family or class reunion, a beach vacation, or another special occasion. The last few years I have competed in the Mrs. Georgia pageant. Last year, I was first runner-up and won the swimsuit segment of the competition. After four kids, that's an accomplishment, if I do say so myself!

I want my body to be in proportion for the pageant. The area that always needs work is my upper thighs. I go on the Fast Track for several weeks, eating lots of vegetables and other healthy carbs. I also step up my exercise program. Transitioning to more vegetables in lieu of complex carbs enables me to be leaner in the thighs. Of course, I ramp up my entire exercise regimen significantly for several weeks before the pageant as well.

I also do a series of cleanses pretty much every spring, including a colonic and a liver/gallbladder cleanse to eliminate fat stored in those organs. Think of them as you do having a regular oil change for your car. After the liver/gallbladder cleanse, I always do a foot ionization detox bath, which draws heavy metals and other toxins out of your body via the bottoms of your feet. I've also used a vibration machine, a platform that oscillates at high frequency, transferring vibrations to your muscles, tendons, and other tissues, thus increasing muscle contractions and burning more energy. Spending time in an infrared sauna helps eliminate still more toxins. I find that these cleanses free up my body to achieve its natural weight and speed up the process.

Colonics and enemas are nothing new. If food goes in, it has to come out. As a culture, we live on processed food, which binds in the bowel and the rest of the body. Unless you are also eating lots of fruits and vegetables, especially those full of roughage, you are in trouble. Add in the environmental toxins accumulating in your body, and it is clear you need to do whatever it takes to clean it out.

Must you have to do a colonic or those other procedures to be successful on the Essential Oils Diet? No. But if you do want to take it to the next level and get even faster or greater success, they are worth considering.

Whether you are going to a reunion or getting ready for that beach visit or whatever, once you are following the Essential Lifestyle, you are just taking it up a notch from what you are doing on a regular basis.

Pre- and Postpartum Meals

Mama Z here. When you're pregnant, you should be eating for one and a half, *not two*. If you do gain excess weight, it is important to realize it will take you longer to transition back to your pre-pregnancy weight. Otherwise, you could become discouraged and wind up retaining all or much of the weight. That needn't happen.

For the first couple of weeks after delivery, I follow the Essential Lifestyle. Then I transition to the Essential Fast Track for four to six weeks to get back to my pre-pregnancy weight. Even if you have a fair amount of weight to lose, don't get stuck following the Fast Track for more than one month. Instead, transition to the Essential Lifestyle. It may take you a bit longer to shed your baby pounds, but you are more likely to keep them off.

So what do I eat? Usually I have a Living Fuel or Mama Z Bio-active Breakfast Shake (page 222) and our Fat-Burning Matcha Latte (page 215) for breakfast. Lunch is a salad, with hard-boiled eggs, tuna, or leftovers from dinner the night before, or an egg-white omelet with lots of veggies. Dinner is more of the same. I always try to make my main dish serve as the "dressing" over a bed of greens. Once I move out of the Fast Track, I eat just a little bit less than I did during pregnancy, and instead of watching my weight go up, I watch it come down naturally.

While you are breastfeeding, your baby is going to get what he needs off the top. As long as you eat the healthy fats found in such foods as avocados and eggs and nutrient-dense leafy greens and other foods in the Essential Oils Diet, there are plenty of calories and nutrients for both of you. However, if you must boost your milk production, also incorporate organic gluten-free oats, breast milk tea, and basil and fennel essential oils.

Getting Back in Shape After Childbirth

Mama Z here. Don't do any abdominal exercises after a vaginal birth for at least two weeks. And even then, just work on the transabdominal muscles underneath the superficial abs. As a small person delivering big babies, my frontal abs have torn each time. This separation of the right and left muscles that hold your tummy flat is called *diastasis recti,* which can also occur during surgery. To get rid of my "mummy tummy," I bind my abs with a loose postpartum wrap—you can easily find these on Amazon—for the first couple of days after birth and then switch to a tighter wrap for a couple of weeks.

Once I am at the point where I can start using my abs again, usually two to six weeks postpartum, I'll switch over to the Tupler Technique, an exercise program designed by Julie Tupler, RN, to rebuild the inner framework of your abs, incorporating the interlocking Diastasis Rehab Splint, which wraps snugly around your waist and tummy. (It doesn't affect how clothes lie on your body as some of the bulky wraps do.) In total, I'll bind my abs for the first six months. Be sure to get clearance from your doctor or midwife before you start to work out your abs.

If you were not into exercise before you had your baby, transition to moderate exercise after a couple of weeks, perhaps just walking for a mile or two a day. It could take you more than four to six weeks to get back to your goal weight. If you live an active lifestyle and are eating the right food, you are going to naturally transition back to the pre-pregnancy weight more quickly.

To help with postpartum stretch marks, I recommend an essential oil blend that incorporates two drops each of lavender, geranium, frankincense, and helichrysum essential oils for every ounce of carrier oil, preferably fractionated coconut or organic jojoba oil; both are relatively watery and able to permeate more deeply into the dermis of the skin. If you have had a C-section, you can use the same essential oils with a wrap to help decrease inflammation, move extra water out of tissues, and tighten and tone the area. I also make a shower gel that has some of these oils in it.

Finally, I use a plastic exfoliator or exfoliating shower gloves with my shower gel to slough off dead skin so new skin can regenerate. So you are tightening, toning, and also healing. Once you make it through the stretch marks and/or scar tissue from a C-section—you'll know when you can run your hands across your abdomen and it doesn't feel weird—you are ready for that next step, which is a muslin and plastic wrap that uses essential oils (see page 276). You will soon be better than back to normal!

POST-SURGERY ESSENTIALS

After an operation, just as with childbirth, allow yourself a transition period. For those first couple of weeks, make sure that you follow the Essential Oils Lifestyle. If being off your feet or unable to exercise has packed on some extra pounds, you can transition to the Fast Track two weeks post-op and stay there for four to six weeks, depending on how much weight you have to shed.

If you have had abdominal surgery, you may want to wear a wrap to hold things in. (See Getting Back in Shape After Childbirth on page 159.) Discuss with your surgeon when you can start to exercise again and which, if any, modifications to make. To minimize scarring, use the same essential oil blend as described for stretch marks. If you have an incision on your body, always talk to your health-care provider to find out when you can begin to use essential oils. If the incision is glued rather than stitched, essential oils will break down the adhesive, so don't use them for at least the first twenty-four to forty-eight hours.

Making Sure Your Kids Are Good to Go

Mama Z here. Following the Essential Lifestyle has to be a family endeavor. Mom and Dad can't eat differently than their kids do. No one wants to cook two or more different meals every day. Such an approach isn't sustainable. Moreover, it sends a confusing message to kids.

When you eat a certain way at home, as we do, clearly you want to see your children eat just as healthfully at preschool, school, or day camp. This is particularly important, of course, if a child has an allergy to peanuts or another food. But it's equally important if she has food sensitivities to dairy, sugar, gluten, and preservatives, as our children do. Even absent a specifc allergy, eating the wrong things can make her life miserable—think constipation, bloating, diarrhea, headaches, nightmares, and other maladies.

We treat our kids' sensitivities the way other people treat allergies. Sometimes we say that they actually have "allergies" so schools, day-care facilities, and summer camps take us seriously. Technically, a sensitivity is an "allergic-type response," so we're not lying, in case you're wondering.

My experience with our three school-age children is that it is perfectly possible to keep them safe away from home. Here's how we do it:

- *Communicate a zero-tolerance policy to the school.* Don't bother distinguishing between food allergies and food sensitivities.
- *Pack lunch at home.* Each child has an insulated lunch bag filled with a sandwich or other meal, a beverage, perhaps a coconut yogurt cup, fruit, and a snack.
- *Provide extra snacks.* I deliver a different bag of snacks for each child, based on his or her needs, to the school. The bag might include organic non-GMO SkinnyPop popcorn, packs of squeezable fruit puree, organic fruit rolls, certain Lärabars, or homemade snacks. I usually replenish supplies three times a year.
- *Celebrate health at birthdays.* On one of our children's birthday, I'll bring healthy cupcakes for the whole class. I always make a big batch and freeze some. I also ask the teacher to keep me apprised of other children's birthdays, so I can send our child off that day with his or her own substitute cupcake.
- *Make it yummy.* The most important thing is to ensure your child's snacks are as delicious and appealing as those the other kids may be eating.

MAMA Z TIP

When your child is invited to a birthday party, call the mom ahead of time and explain that he or she has food allergies. Ask what she is planning to serve and offer to bring your healthy equivalent.

TRANSITIONING KIDS TO A HEALTHIER DIET

Mama Z here. If you've changed your way of eating, you'll want to make it a family affair. Gluten, sugar, and dairy are the top three agents that cause inflammatory and allergic responses. How do you move your children from whatever they're eating now to a healthier diet? A doctor I discussed this with years ago told me, "When people are on Oreos, I get them to move to Newman-Os first, then move them on to something healthier."

It's a *transitional* process. So if your kids are eating sugar-laden cereal for breakfast, move to a similar organic cereal with no added sugar. Substitute organic almond or coconut milk for cow's milk, and stevia or honey crystals instead of sugar. Top it with sliced banana or blueberries.

The next step would be to introduce variety in the form of green shakes and eggs. (See page 210 for more breakfast ideas.) Fortunately, the younger a child, the easier it is to retrain her taste buds away from sugar. Even kids who say they hate vegetables usually like raw carrots and celery with a tasty dip. Finally, make dessert a sometime thing, not a daily expectation. Overall, make food fun. Among the many bonuses of such an approach is that your kids will grow up with a level of awareness about how to be healthy that is missing in so many adults today.

Leaving for College—and Eating Healthy

Mama Z here. Say you're heading off to college—or have a child going away to school—and you want to keep eating as well as you have been at home. You certainly don't want to gain the dreaded "freshman fifteen" that so many people pack on during their first year in college. Residential colleges require that you purchase a meal plan so you're likely to be eating most of your meals in the cafeteria. If you are lucky, there are options for people who are vegetarians or vegans, or who avoid gluten or dairy products. Some might even have a policy of using organic produce. But don't count on it. You may have to thread your way carefully through the food stations.

- *Bone up before you go.* Hopefully, you know your way around a kitchen. If you aren't already cooking some of your own meals, take some "lessons" from the family's chief cook and bottle washer so that you can put together a simple meal. That way, you'll have some alternatives when none of the offerings in the cafeteria appeal.
- *Head for the salad bar.* Your best options will be here. Top a mixed salad with some grilled salmon or halibut.
- *Look for an omelet station.* If you find one, you're in luck. Ask for an egg-white or whole-egg omelet with spinach or other veggies cooked in butter or olive oil. No omelet station? Make your own over a hot plate in your room.
- *Check out the dorm.* Some have kitchenettes with a fridge and a stove, although a microwave is more likely.
- *Stock up on healthy snacks.* That way, when you can't face another meal in the cafeteria, you have options.
- *Be smart when you eat out.* Part of the college experience is joining new friends to go out for pizza. Make the best choice you can under the circumstances.

MAMA Z TIP

Don't wait until your child is heading off to college to talk to him about healthy food and show him how to prepare a few simple dishes.

Detoxing as a Way of Life

We hope that your first month on the Fast Track and this introduction to the Essential Lifestyle have sensitized you to your body's messaging system. If you ignore warning signs such as feeling toxic, empty, always on the verge of illness, unfocused, and continually tired, you can lose the crucial connection with your body. You may be on the way to becoming your own toxic waste dump, suffering from out-of-whack hormones and chronic inflammation, putting you at serious risk for serious diseases.

Constant exposure to environmental toxins compounds such a condition and increases the possibility of chronic disease, as well as surplus pounds. We'll discuss those important connections and how you can detox your body in the following chapter.

CHAPTER 8

STAYING HEALTHY IN A TOXIC WORLD: A GUIDE TO BEATING ENVIRONMENTAL TOXINS

"Your body is a richly nuanced intuitive receiver."

—JUDITH ORLOFF, MD

Food and physical activity are critical to staying healthy and slim, but alone they are simply not enough to ensure permanent and glowing health. The challenge we face is enjoying a healthy lifestyle in an increasingly toxic world. So, we're going to take a deep dive into a number of other factors that influence your health and ability to live an abundant life, from electronic devices to water quality, cleaning products, and more.

Big-picture transformation ultimately is the theme of this book. Now that we have dealt with the eight healthy habits discussed in chapter 5 (page 93) and the Essential Lifestyle strategies and tips in chapter 7, we also want to make you aware of other significant factors that can negatively impact your health. Our objective is not to scare you, but rather to give you a road map with which to navigate this complicated world of toxic threats by either avoiding them or replacing them with healthier alternatives. You'll also learn how some of our modern "conveniences" play a role in obesity and the rise of chronic diseases such as diabetes.

Just one example: Conventional laundry products expose your body—and those of your family—to a host of chemicals. Trust us, those cleaning agents do *not* wash away during the rinse cycle. Don't believe us? You can smell the proof well after you take clothes out of the washer and dryer. Unless your laundry products are scented with pure essential oils—and most are not—synthetic fragrances full of toxic ingredients are transferred to your skin and remain glued there all day long, every day of the week, year after year after year. Scary, yes, but the reality is that you can get your clothes just as clean using safe, natural ingredients, including some with essential oils.

To watch a five-part video tour of our home, where we show you how we've given our kitchen, pantry, laundry room, bathroom, and garden a complete toxic-free health makeover, visit EssentialOilsDiet.com.

Dr. Z here. When I became a Christian in 2003, my mentor at the time said, "Eric, your body is the temple of the Holy Spirit and you need to take care of it. That means more than just what you are eating; it means what you are putting on your skin. It is what you are inhaling and the environment in which you put your body."

Mama Z here. The air and water around you, the devices you plug into your wall, the items in your kitchen and bathroom, all make a difference. Unbeknownst to us, our first house had toxic black mold, so we know what it's like to live in a bad environment. We also now know what it's like to live in a healthy environment, although it took us a number of years to achieve it. Our home is now a vibrant place with great energy for our friends, family, and anyone else who enters. We want to bless you by sharing that knowledge.

God designed you so that fevers, stomachaches, rashes, and headaches serve as clues and warning signs of challenges to your body's natural balance. Today, however, these natural red flags can be masked with makeup, prescription medications, supplements, and even essential oils! When used to treat a symptom without addressing the root cause, they all become Band-Aids.

Is it better to banish the evidence of acne or skin rashes or eliminate the body's natural responses to acid reflux or leaky gut than to acknowledge these "signals" as warnings that something is wrong? Of course not! Treating symptoms rather than addressing root causes mutes your innate ability to listen to your body's warnings.

Don't Let Technology Control You

When most people think about toxins in their home, they envision allergens in the air, chemicals in cleaning products, preservatives in processed foods, or heavy metals such as lead in paint. Yes, all of these are toxic and should be avoided, but what about the undetectable toxins that technology emits via the airwaves all day long?

Technology has changed our everyday lives in profound ways. No one wants to give up shopping online, accessing limitless sources of information, or tele-chatting with friends and family hundreds or thousands of miles away. But technology also has a darker side. Remember, convenience never comes without a cost.

What will be the long-term impact of the tech revolution on our bodies and brains? And how about the effects from decades of eating genetically modified food blasted with pesticides? You could say that we are all guinea pigs caught in a confluence of such "laboratory experiments." If you are concerned about your health and that of your loved ones, until the results of these experiments are known, the wisest approach is to err on the side of caution. To do that, we advise you to eliminate or at least moderate as many of these dangerous influences as possible.

Our objective is to take some control of technology, instead of letting it control us. From the time your cell phone awakens you in the morning until you send your last text message of the day or turn off your television, technology is controlling your brain, altering your hormonal cycle, and even affecting your ability to lose weight, among other negatives.

We are in the same situation as everyone else: we get freaked out by all this stuff, but we don't want to live in fear. One of our favorite Bible verses says, "You don't have the spirit of fear, but of power, love and a sound mind" *(2 Timothy 1:7)*. The bottom line is that despite knowing that all this technology is not good for your body and your brain, at this point it is unavoidable. Some people say, "Just chill out and live with it." We strongly disagree. Fortunately, there are ways you can wrest control away from these devices. So our two-pronged approach is first, don't panic; second, take preventive and defensive action.

First let's address electromagnetic fields (EMFs), which come from electronic and other electrical devices that affect the behavior of objects, including us, in their space. (Your body has its own electrical system, so EMFs can mess with *your* wiring.) Microwave ovens and cell phones are two major offenders, but you'll learn about some others as well. In each case, we'll talk about how to corral EMFs.

Microwave Ovens: Weigh Convenience vs. Risk

We have been seduced by the shiny apple of convenience to do harmful things to ourselves. The microwave oven is a perfect example. We guarantee that your great-grandma and all your grandmas before her lived without one. In the thirteen years we have been married, we have increasingly moved to natural ways of doing everything in order to minimize environmental risks to our family. We live happily without a microwave, and so can you. Yes, it is convenient, but is the convenience worth the risk?

Bottom line: You need to detox your life. Deep-sixing your microwave is just one step.

Electromagnetic Exposure

So, what exactly are the health risks posed by a microwave oven? No, we're not talking about chemicals in plastic dishes leaching into your food. Using PBA-free plastic or, better yet, glass dishes has resolved that concern. Nor is there any conclusive evidence that microwaving food changes its molecular structure. It is the actual wireless signals—the microwaves themselves, meaning the EMFs, which are a form of low-level radiation—that are the subject of our concern.

Microwave ovens use the same wireless technology that powers remote controls, radios, walkie-talkies, cell phones, baby monitors, Bluetooth devices, computers, and Wi-Fi routers. All use EMFs classified as low level, but microwave ovens are among the devices that use the highest frequency EMFs that can still be considered low level.[1]

To date, there is no smoking gun proving that using a microwave oven has directly caused a disease, but what we *don't* know about EMFs could harm us. In one study, extremely low frequency electromagnetic fields have been shown to fragment DNA in pregnant animals, which could have detrimental effects on fertility and embryo development.[2] Why would you want to put your genetic code at risk for mere convenience? In fact, multiple research trials have shown that electromagnetic fields can have destructive effects on fetal development, gonadal function, sex hormones, and pregnancy.[3]

We can make good decisions only if we have good information, but at this time the *full* impact of EMFs on human health is largely a question mark. However, many studies do conclusively verify an increased risk of several forms of cancer,[4] diabetes,[5] and even weight gain.[6] Overexposure to low-level EMFs has also been shown to produce a horrifying list of other health problems. We're talking sleep disorders, headaches, fatigue, dysesthesia, concentration and attention dysfunction, memory changes, dizziness, irritability, restlessness and anxiety, nausea, skin burning and tingling, and EEG (electroencephalogram) changes.[7]

Why would anyone want to play around with any of these conditions in order to save a few minutes in the kitchen? After reading this terrifying list, we suspect that you'll agree.

The same also applies to long-term exposure to microwave radiation from radar and mobile communication systems.[8] Try to avoid living near electrical and telephone towers and sleeping next to your Wi-Fi routers at all cost. More on that on page 175.

Cell Phones and Your Health

No one wants to live without them—and that includes us—but cell phones pose a number of health risks that center around EMFs. Again, there are ways to minimize their impact.

- **The cancer question.** According to the World Health Organization, your cell phone emits EMFs a thousand times stronger than those of the base stations that transmit the radio waves. Although brain cancers in children have increased in recent years, studies have not yet found a clear link between brain cancer and cell phone use. However, the International Agency for Research on Cancer has described the EMFs produced by cell phones as *possibly* carcinogenic to humans.[9] Because it could take up to twenty-five years for a tumor to develop, and most people have not been using cell phones that long, long-term research is unavailable. That means we are effectively flying blind.

- **The evidence is in.** One study did show that glioma, a rare form of brain cancer, is three times more prevalent in individuals who had used a cell phone for twenty-five years compared with those who had used one for less than a year.[10] Another study showed a correlation between being right-handed or left-handed and the parallel location of a brain tumor, suggesting that holding a cell phone to one side of your head could be a factor.[11] In fact, one-sided cell phone use has been linked to a two and a half times increased risk of developing a brain tumor on that side of your head![12]

    There *is* a clear link between cell phone use and sleep disorders—EMF transmissions disrupt production of the sleep hormone melatonin,[13] a risk factor for being overweight. Cell phone radiation can make red blood cells seep hemoglobin, leading to heart complications.[14] It also decreases sperm count and damages sperm DNA.[15] Long-term exposure to EMFs can also impair hearing.[16]

Cell Phone Myths

It turns out that using a hands-free device isn't much safer than a handheld one. Nor is using a wireless headset, which actually increases your exposure to EMFs. You have probably seen various protective plates, shields, and other such devices advertised, but it is doubtful that any are effective. *How* you use your phone is actually more significant than your phone's SAR (specific absorption rate) level.[17] This is the amount of radio frequency absorbed by your body, which should not exceed 1.6 watts per kilogram. (You can find this rating in your phone's instruction manual or at FCC.gov/general/specific-absorption-rate-sar-cellular-telephones.)

Sensible Cell Phone Use

To minimize your exposure to EMFs, use your cell phone only when necessary. Having a landline is an added expense, but it does mean you can reduce or eliminate outgoing mobile calls at home. Here are some other defensive strategies:

- *Keep the phone away from your head.* At a 2-inch distance, the signal is roughly a quarter of the original strength. Four inches diminishes it to one-sixteenth. Better yet, use the speaker mode whenever possible. Or use a safe handset such as the wired ear buds that came with the phone. *Wireless* headsets expose you to still more EMFs.
- *Adjust your settings.* When not in use, put your phone on flight mode, which turns off the wireless transmitter, reducing EMF exposure. Or just turn it off or set it to other preferences. (See Foil Blue Light on page 177.)
- *Text instead of calling* whenever possible, but don't hold the phone in your lap as you text.
- *Avoid areas with a weak signal* such as basements, elevators, and parking garages, which can cause your phone to emit up

to one thousand times more radiation. Instead, go outside whenever possible.

- *Use a stationary location.* In a moving car or train, the phone is constantly scanning for the nearest cell tower to contact, increasing EMF emissions.
- *Use a cell phone pouch,* aka a pocket shield, rather than a phone case. A conventional case can block the antenna so the phone actually has to work harder, emitting more EMFs, to receive a signal. Two brands that do a good job are RF Safe (RFSafe .com/product-category/phone-radiation-safety/rf-safe-pocket -shields) and Less EMF (LessEMF.com/cellphone.html).
- *Hold the phone away from you after dialing.* Wait until you hear the recipient answer before bringing it closer to your body. Again, the phone emits more radiation when trying to connect. With an incoming call, extend the phone until you hear the other party.
- *If you must carry the phone with you,* place the keypad side closer to your body with the back facing out to angle the EMFs away from you. Again, never carry a cell phone in your pocket.
- *Never sleep beside your cell phone.* At the very least, put it on airplane mode and turn off the Wi-Fi before you go to bed. Charge it elsewhere. If you must be reachable at all times, keep it on the other side of the room. Better yet, have a landline phone next to your bed.

Dr. Z here. I used to carry my cell phone in a holster, but it got hot, just as the phone does if you keep it next to your ear too long. Think about what that is doing to your whole body. But people are in love with their phone. It is always with them, and they are always touching it. This thing is not your friend. Rather, it is a tool, a means to an end, and a highly dangerous one at that. I also used a wireless headset until my ear started burning and the headpieces gave me vertigo or buzzing in my ear. These headsets use Bluetooth technology, which concentrates EMFs in your ear and your brain. I switched to normal headphones, although I know that the magnets in them mean they are not a perfect solution. But at least my ears don't get hot, buzz, or ring anymore.

Wi-Fi and Bluetooth Are Unavoidable

Wi-Fi and Bluetooth technology also emit EMFs, presenting yet another hazard, and the higher the gigahertz (GHz), meaning the speed of the processor, the greater the threat to your health. Today, so many devices use the 2.4 GHz band that it has become overloaded, resulting in dropped connections and slowed speeds. The 5 GHz band is less congested and provides higher speeds and more stable connections. But there is concern in some quarters that when we get up to 10 GHz, it could change our DNA. Still, it seems the movement to higher gigahertz is inevitable.

As long as your router is on, your Wi-Fi is operative, sending out EMFs. Best to turn it off at night. At the very least, make sure your router is nowhere near the bedrooms so that it is not interfering with sleep. While we are short on research, it is hard to ignore anecdotal evidence—for example, that infants are very sensitive to Wi-Fi. Some friends of ours had a baby with a lot of issues. He couldn't sleep at night and cried on and on. But when the parents turned off the router, disabling the Wi-Fi, he slept soundly. It was that simple. Now they turn it off every night. This is one reason why we limit our older kids' use of their cell phones or tablets in their rooms.

We also simply turn off the Bluetooth function in our cell phones, tablets, computers, and laptops. The only exceptions are when we're using wireless speakers to watch a movie in surround sound or want to talk on the phone hands-free while one of us is driving.

Dr. Z here. Fasting isn't limited to food—we recommend technology fasts, too. You have to be in control of technology or it is going to control you. Our family takes a tech break on certain days. For example, when I took our three older kids to Disney World for a week, no one used his or her iPad. They played board games and built things with their Legos, but there was no screen time—nada—and they did just fine.

ARE YOU ADDICTED TO YOUR CELL PHONE?

Dr. Z here. When you post on Facebook or another social media site, how many times do you check to see who liked it or commented on your post? Such a habit can become a compulsion. In fact, the notification sound triggers a dopamine response in the brain, just as cocaine does. Cell phones are even more addictive than crack, according to author and TED speaker Simon Sineck, who asserts that kids can become addicted to their phone by the time they are ten.[18]

That is what happened to me, although I didn't realize it initially. Whenever I found notifications, whether from Facebook or another social media site, e-mail, or whatever, I had to go to it. I do most of my work on the phone, and I had become totally addicted to both work and my cell phone. Once I realized my problem, my solution to eliminating the clutter was to turn off Notifications (under Settings) on my mobile. After I did this, I was able to peel myself away from the screen much more easily!

I do leave text messages on so that I can see if Mama Z needs me. Now the only way I know whether or not someone else is trying to contact me is if I go into e-mail, Facebook, Twitter, or any other app on my phone. If you leave notifications on, all of those little red numbers—and there's a reason they are red—scream at you whenever you go to your home screen. I have none of that now and have regained some measure of control over technology.

I challenge you to show me a family eating at a restaurant these days without youngsters glued to their devices. Of course, adults often model this behavior for them.

Foil Blue Light

We mentioned "blue light" briefly in chapter 5, but now let's delve a little deeper. Blue wavelengths are emitted by the sun, which is why they boost attention, reaction times, and mood, all of which are beneficial during the day but disruptive at night. Also emitted by televisions, computers, cell phones, other electronic devices, and even LED lightbulbs, blue light has similar effects to those of EMFs. Both interfere with the production of melatonin, known as the sleep hormone,[19] which normally occurs as darkness falls and explains why you should avoid exposure to blue light two to three hours before bedtime.

You already know that sleep disturbances can prompt weight gain and interfere with weight-loss efforts. But melatonin plays another important role: It destroys the free radicals implicated in cancer, heart disease, and many other diseases. Low melatonin levels are associated with a number of different forms of cancer.[20]

You don't want blue light razzing with your brain and keeping you awake at night, which will affect your ability to experience the abundant life, attain your natural weight, and enjoy vibrant health. And you certainly don't want to make yourself more susceptible to serious diseases. The obvious answer is not to use such devices in the evening; however, this isn't practical for most people.

Because your eyes have low sensitivity to blue wavelengths, your smartphone increases the light intensity at night, which boosts electricity use and the level of electromagnetic fields generated by its displays.[21,22] That's why you should change the settings on your mobile device or otherwise counteract blue light. Here's how:

- Use the Night Shift setting under Display & Brightness on your cell phone. It blocks the blue light with an amber filter. Simply set the times you want this to go into effect in the evening and end in the morning.
- A low-tech but effective option is to wear amber-tinted glasses, which block the effects of blue light on melatonin

production.[23] You can order a pair for under $10 from Amazon and other online retailers.

- Download free software for your PC or Mac, as well as for tablets and cell phones, from f.lux (JustGetFlux.com), which gives your screen an amber cast after dusk. You can adjust the settings to suit the season and your bedtime. Or simply turn on the Night Shift setting under System Preferences.

The Usual Suspects

While technology poses a whole megillah of challenges to our health and well-being, other threats have been around for a while, which is not to diminish their dangers. Many folks either ignore them or think there is not much they can do about water quality, air quality, toxic garden and landscape products, insecticides, endocrine disruptors, and other harmful chemicals in our homes, including those in body-care products. We beg to differ. Let's look briefly at the issues surrounding each of these problematic areas and provide you with workable solutions to dramatically lighten your toxic load.

Toxins in the Water Supply

Like a plant, without water you would wither and die. Water is essential for life, but pure water is increasingly difficult to come by. The lead in the public water supply of Flint, Michigan, has gotten a lot of well-deserved press, but it is only the most visible example of the crisis facing the nation's water supply. In addition to old lead piping, which can leach lead into the water, agrichemicals, such as glyphosate-based herbicides (GBHs), enter groundwater, underground aquifers, and municipal water supplies nearly everywhere on earth.

- Drinking-water nitrate levels *within* the regulatory limit are associated with greater risk of both colon cancer and neural tube defects.[24]

- Atrazine and nitrate, even at levels that are well below the legal limits for drinking water, are associated with very preterm delivery, a serious danger to both newborns and mothers.[25]
- Prenatal nitrate exposure from drinking water *at EPA-acceptable levels* can cause spina bifida, limb deficiency, cleft palate, cleft lip, neural tube defects, central nervous system defects, musculoskeletal defects, and congenital heart defect.[26]
- Nitrate in drinking water is associated with bladder cancer.[27]
- Glyphosate-based herbicides are the most commonly used herbicides worldwide and are found in groundwater, bottled water, and in the urine of farm workers (even when used below the recommended limits).[28,29,30,31,32,33]

Pathogens in drinking water also cause a wide range of extremely uncomfortable to outright deadly diseases such as gastroenteritis (vibrios, *E. coli*), cholera (*Vibrio cholerae*), typhoid fever (salmonella), protozoan infection (giardiasis, cryptosporidiosis), and bacillary (shigella) or amoebic dysentery.[34] Thanks to the nature of their construction and active interventions, modern improved water sources should be free of outside contamination. This offers some degree of protection but cannot guarantee the water is free of fecal matter, and water safety is not consistent among sources.[35] Fungal contaminants often resist treatment and form a biofilm with bacteria and protozoa, making all three nearly impossible to kill.[36] Even treated water in developed countries frequently makes people acutely ill![37]

Even if you have your own well, your water could be tainted. It could also contain bacteria, silt, sediment, and chemicals such as chlorine. Plus, you simply don't know what is in your pipes, especially in an older house. To counteract these problems, we installed a whole-house water filtration system. It's reassuring to know the water in the shower or tub has been scrubbed of toxins.

Underneath the kitchen sink, we installed a reverse osmosis system as well to ensure the water is 100 percent pure before touching our lips. Less expensive units simply sit on the counter beside the sink. A dual system addresses both the water source and any toxins in pipes.

The Environmental Working Group (EWG) provides a database of public water-supply companies. To find out which toxins might be flowing from your taps, go to EWG.org/tapwater and click on your state. If you have a well, your local government should be able to direct you to a reliable laboratory that tests water quality.

The Question of Air Quality

Consider this shocking fact: According to the EWG, the air inside a home is somewhere between two and five times more polluted than the air outside.[38] Artificial fragrances and other chemicals in household products, body-care products, and even air fresheners contribute to this toxic stew. Get in the driver's seat by simply not buying certain items. Instead, make your own, following the recipes in *The Healing Power of Essential Oils*. There are also responsible companies that make products we can recommend with confidence, which you can find at NaturalLivingFamily.com/how-to-be-healthy/.

Additionally, products such as paint, synthetic carpeting, vinyl flooring, and mandated flame-retardant building products that are a fact of modern life off-gas long after application or installation. If you are remodeling, choose safer products whenever possible. At the very least, allow the house to air out after painting, refinishing floors, or installing new flooring. Another major source of indoor toxins is the off-gassing from the foam used in most upholstered furniture, including mattresses. (The Environmental Working Group suggests alternative products at EWG.org/healthyhomeguide.)

Other polluted air can obviously enter your house whenever you open a door or window. Legislation eliminating the use of leaded gasoline has cleaned up our air somewhat, but forest fires, smog, industrial farming, and coal-fired power plants still produce plenty of pollution. A whole-house filtration system can help minimize exterior sources of air pollution. (See Detox Resources on page 334.) If you cannot afford such a system, there are some relatively inexpensive portable products available.

Toxins in Your Yard

Unless you or your lawn service is using 100 percent organic products, chances are that your lawn has been treated with chemical fertilizers, pesticides, herbicides, and other toxic lawn-care products. If you are growing veggies in soil full of such products, residues of those poisons turn up in your meals and tummy. Children are particularly sensitive to these contaminates. Pesticides also alter hormones, stimulating weight gain, among other effects.[39,40]

Farmers and homeowners alike use hundreds of millions of pounds of pesticides and insecticides around homes, gardens, and farms annually, including well-known and heavily marketed products such as glyphosate-based herbicides, including Roundup. Exposure to these toxins has been linked to numerous conditions from eye and skin irritation to cancer, birth defects, and neurodevelopmental disorders.[41,42,43] Fertilizers such as Miracle-Gro also contain toxins. This is bad enough in your garden, but wind wafts residues into your house and feet track them in, contaminating the air and surfaces.

In our garden, we use only natural nontoxic and organic products such as bonemeal, earthworm casings, and essential oils. Blood meal is a great source of nitrogen, and as an added benefit, it deters rabbits and other critters eager to nibble your veggies. Diatomaceous earth banishes crawling insects and other pests.

If you give plants a good start in life, they won't need a chemical boost. When planting, we use a good organic fertilizer, such as Sure Start or Dr. Earth, which helps roots develop quickly. We also use a natural weed and grass killer made with essential oils. Natural insecticides, fungicides, and miticides are safe to use on both your garden and your houseplants. Among other brand names we recommend are Garden Safe—they make a fungicide based on neem oil—Nature's Care, EcoSMART, EcoScraps, and Jobe's Organics. Of course, aged compost is also a healthy addition to soil.

To watch how we've given our garden a complete toxic-free health makeover, visit EssentialOilsDiet.com.

Kill Bugs, Not Humans

Dr. Z here. While we are on the subject of bugs, let's talk about insect repellents. The Environmental Protection Agency (EPA) estimates that each year one-third of Americans use a product that contains DEET (N, N-diethyl-meta-toluamide) to repel mosquitos, ticks, and other biting insects that transmit disease. Although the EPA claims that DEET "does not present a health concern," a study of National Parks employees required to use it on the job found that a full 25 percent of them experienced effects attributed to DEET. These included abnormal sweating, nausea, headaches, dizziness, difficulty concentrating, skin irritation and rashes, and numb or burning lips.[44]

Studies on rats have found that frequent and prolonged exposure to DEET kills brain cells and causes behavioral changes. The authors concluded that people should avoid products that contain it.[45,46] It's worth noting that DEET has been chemically engineered *not* to deteriorate for twelve hours after application, meaning it remains on your body long after you likely no longer need protection. Why use a product that contains DEET when essential oil formulations can be just as effective?

Mama Z here. One of my favorite essential oils for summer is peppermint. We live near Atlanta—there's a reason natives call it "Hot-lanta"!—and when I water the plants, I apply peppermint oil to my body to cool down. Years ago I used a brand that wasn't very strong. Then I got one that was "real" peppermint oil, meaning it wasn't adulterated. It was the middle of summer, but when I put it on my body, I felt like I had gone to the Arctic. That's how I learned the importance of dilution, especially with peppermint oil. But the bugs wouldn't touch me with a ten-foot pole!

MAMA Z TIP

To avoid ant invasions, put a drop of peppermint essential oil and a little bit of coconut oil on a cotton ball and wipe it around the inside of the door frame to act as a barrier.

Dangerous Food Additives

Hard to believe, but more than ten thousand food additives, including pesticides, are permitted in our food supply. There is obviously no way to avoid all of them; however, eating only organic food and reading labels carefully allows you to avoid many of them. The EWG has created a Healthy Living app that allows you to scan the UPC code on a food (or a cosmetic or a household product) to see a list of ingredients. As a general rule of thumb, if you cannot pronounce it or don't recognize it as food, an ingredient is likely to be an additive or preservative. Our advice is simple: Put the product back on the shelf.

To help you navigate your way through this culinary maze, EWG has come up with a Shopper's Guide to Pesticides in Produce, consisting of two lists: the Dirty Dozen (page 184) and the Clean Fifteen (page 185), which it updates annually. The first lists the conventionally grown produce most likely to be contaminated with pesticides;

the second, produce least likely to be so. If you can't buy all organic produce, these lists help you understand which fruits and vegetables should absolutely be organic (or avoided) and which you are relatively safe buying that are conventionally grown. These two lists, which are updated annually, can also be downloaded in a convenient wallet- or cell-phone-size format at EWG.org/foodnews.

THE DIRTY DOZEN

From the top down, the following conventionally grown fruits and vegetables are the most heavily treated with pesticides:

1. Strawberries
2. Spinach
3. Nectarines
4. Apples
5. Grapes
6. Peaches
7. Cherries
8. Pears
9. Tomatoes
10. Celery
11. Potatoes
12. Sweet bell peppers

The Far-Reaching Effects of Endocrine Disruptors

We've mentioned on several occasions that estrogen-like chemicals known as endocrine disruptors can promote weight gain—basically, your body thinks you're pregnant!—diabetes, and other metabolic diseases, but that's just the tip of the iceberg. They can also wreak all sorts of other hormonal havoc, playing a role in female cancers, prostate cancer in men, and thyroid problems.

From the top down, the following conventionally grown fruits and vegetables are the least contaminated with pesticides:

1. Avocados
2. Sweet corn
3. Pineapples
4. Cabbages
5. Onions
6. Sweet peas
7. Papayas
8. Asparagus
9. Mangoes
10. Eggplants
11. Honeydew melons
12. Kiwis
13. Cantaloupes
14. Cauliflower
15. Broccoli

So where do hormone disruptors live? The short answer is everywhere. You probably know that they are found in most plastics, including most bottled water bottles and the thin film of plastic that lines most canned foods. They lurk in preservatives and stabilizing agents such as BHT (butylated hydroxytoluene) in waffles, bread, crackers, cooking oils, and almost all processed foods. Most cosmetics and sunscreens contain parabens, another estrogen-like compound. Anything with artificial flavoring, color, or fragrance contains endocrine disruptors, including laundry detergent and most cleaning products. Ditto for most toothpastes, mouthwashes, and hand sanitizers. Add anything made with phthalates, which soften plastic, ranging from plastic wrap to rubber gloves and vinyl flooring. This list could go on for pages, but you've got the picture.

How is this possible? Believe it or not, there are no safety standards or testing data required before a household cleaning product can be marketed. The average household contains hundreds of toxic chemicals, ranging from synthetic fragrances to the noxious fumes in oven cleaners. While each exposure may be minute, chronic exposure adds to the number of chemicals stored in your body's tissues at a given time, what is called your "toxic load." No wonder you feel heavy sometimes!

How do you avoid these ubiquitous substances and reduce your toxic load? The short answer is to follow the Essential Oils Diet. By eating fresh, organic foods and eliminating almost all processed foods filled with artificial colors, flavors, preservatives, and stabilizers from your diet, you're already well on your way. Now take it to the next step, using our easy-to-do recipes for DIY body-care products for toothpaste, facial cleansers, hand soap and sanitizers, bath salts, mouthwash, and many more. You can find these in *The Healing Power of Essential Oils*. Ditto for our bathroom cleaner, dish soap, dusting spray, glass cleaner, air fresheners, and more cleaning concoctions. Once more, welcome to the fragrant, safe world of essential oils!

To watch a five-part video tour of our home where we show you how we've given our kitchen, bathroom, pantry, laundry room, and garden a complete toxic-free makeover, visit EssentialOilsDiet.com.

Toxic-Free Healthy Home Makeover

The sheer number of areas in which toxins have invaded our homes and lifestyles can seem overwhelming, but keep your cool. As we said earlier, it has taken us years to create an environment as toxin-free as possible. Hopefully, our advice will make it easier for you, but also accept the fact that this is a process. Concentrate on the low-hanging fruit first, perhaps by changing settings on your cell phone, bidding farewell to your microwave, and eliminating problematic foods from your pantry. The last thing we want to do is to create more stress in your life.

To that end, the next and final chapter addresses emotional balance, which along with six other factors is key to good health and an abundant life. Then we'll move on to our delicious recipes and healing remedies using essential oils formulated to help you lose weight, as well as our exercise plan.

CHAPTER 9

THE KEYS TO AN ABUNDANT LIFE

"The thief comes in the night only to steal and destroy; I
come that they may have life and have it abundantly."

—JOHN 10:10

*T*rue abundance is achieved when each of the seven key areas of
your life is balanced and thriving: the emotional, mental, spiritual,
physical, financial, occupational, and social, all of which are intercon-
nected. If your physical body isn't functioning as it should, it's going
to weigh you down mentally and cause strain in your relationships. If
you're not happy in your job or not living up to your full potential,
it's going to impact your emotions, as well as your financial health. If
you're not rooted and grounded spiritually, you will be shipwrecked
by life's storms, and you will suffer from mental and emotional duress.

Like a chain, you are only as strong as your weakest link, which
is why we have found that true transformation starts with having a
mind-set of abundance. Abundance is about finding balance in all aspects of your life as you seek to improve each area without letting
another lag behind. Otherwise, when the going gets tough—and trust
us, it will—you will struggle to develop the lifelong healthy habits
that we've covered thus far because at least one of the seven areas will
inevitably bog you down. Each area of your life falls into one (or more)
of these categories, and your goal is to master every discipline. The
principles of the abundant life promote what we also refer to as biblical
health.

True abundance means that you have your life in order and are content, not lacking for any good thing, as the Bible says *(Psalm 34:10).*

True abundance also means that you have wonderful (and mutually beneficial) relationships with the people in your life, you experience a thriving spiritual connection with God, your emotions are controlled and balanced, you sincerely enjoy the time that you spend earning a living, and your mind and body are healthy and strong. And, of course, *true* abundance means that you're not burdened by debt and that you have more than enough money to live a comfortable life.

In this chapter, we're going to cover five of these seven key areas of life in more detail and outline some easy-to-implement tips on how to find balance and abundance in each area.

Emotional Abundance

Emotional abundance is none other than joy and happiness. When the Bible refers to people as "blessed," it means that they are enviable, fortunate, and, most importantly, happy. In fact, the Hebrew word *esher* and the Greek term *makarios,* meaning "blessed," are used interchangeably with the word *happy* throughout. The Book of Proverbs offers plenty of sage advice on how to achieve an emotionally abundant life. Among the timeless keys to happiness are being at peace with others and with ourselves, finding wisdom in our day-to-day activities with people and at work, thinking before speaking, and guarding our hearts against unforgiveness and bitterness.

"Watch over your heart with all diligence, for from it flow the springs of life" *(Proverbs 4:23)*. You have it in you to be happy. Positive psychology, which uses effective interventions to help individuals, families, and communities thrive, suggests that half of our happiness level is determined by genetics; another 40 percent by our intentional actions; and a mere 10 percent by circumstances such as income, social status, place of residence, and age.[1] Trust us, your ability to be happy is completely within your control!

According to the first World Happiness Report published in 2012, when compared with those who live in the saddest nations, the happiest nations—Norway, Denmark, Iceland, and Switzerland—have average incomes forty times higher and a healthy life expectancy of twenty-eight more years. Citizens of the happiest nations are also much more likely to have someone to call on in times of trouble and to have a sense of freedom, and less likely to perceive widespread corruption in business and government.[2] The happiest countries are generally those where people have their own internal standards, are satisfied in their work, and neither social competition nor excessive materialism are present. Perhaps that is why the United States ranks fourteenth in the most recent World Happiness Report.[3] Interestingly, once basic needs are met, money has little to do with happiness.

Strong, healthy social relationships are the one common denominator of all the happiest places. Other contributing factors include satisfaction with your life, engaging in activities you love, loving other people, using your skills, continually learning, curbing anger and negativity, and having life goals that are bigger than yourself. Also considered important are having more green space and short work commutes.

Reduce Toxic Emotions

When you read about pesticides and the other toxins in chapter 8, you may have not considered some all-too-familiar toxins: those in your heart and mind. Emotional detoxing is as essential as the other types of cleansing we have discussed earlier.

It's natural to have both positive and negative emotions, but when we can't properly manage the negative ones, we can find ourselves in a downward spiral. This can have a serious impact on every aspect of our lives, and especially our health and ability to achieve and maintain one's ideal weight. Just as chemicals can build up in your body, causing a toxic overload, negative emotions can accumulate, torpedoing your relationships, career, overall stress levels, and your body. An emotional-healing detox can help you regain control of your life and achieve mental and emotional balance and, eventually, happiness. Who doesn't want to get the most out of life?

If you are feeling angry, bitter, hurt, discouraged, resentful, regretful, shameful, sorrowful, powerless, or any combination of the above, you need to detox yourself of such feelings. According to Johns Hopkins psychiatrist Karen Swartz, MD, such ongoing emotional states can weaken your immune system and over time increase the risk of depression, heart disease, diabetes, and other diseases.[4] Regular emotional-healing detox breaks will help you get a handle on your emotions and cleanse your entire system so that you can reach your full potential and enjoy the abundant life. Try our Twelve-Step Detox below.

THE TWELVE-STEP DETOX

1. *Let it go.* Forgive those who have wronged you and your entire outlook on life can change, along with an improvement in your physical, mental, and emotional health.[5,6] The past is the past, and no amount of regret can change that.

2. *Release yourself as well.* Having a self-forgiving attitude is indicative of fewer mood disturbances and a better quality of life.[7] Once you forgive others, it's easier to forgive yourself and eliminate guilt and shame. Instead, focus on the future and achieving your full potential. (Sounds like transformation, right?)

3. *Practice self-love.* Instead of hating yourself because you don't meet some unrealistic standard of looks, income, social status, intelligence, or whatever, love yourself as you are. Doing so can make you more able to acknowledge errors and be less hurt by criticism.[8]

4. *Recite positive affirmations.* Specific statements break the cycle of negative thinking and help you visualize change. Here are some of our favorites from the Bible:
   - "I serve an awesome God who promises no evil will befall me and no plague will come near my dwelling." *(Psalm 91:10)*
   - "I serve a faithful God who promises to never leave me nor forsake me." *(Deuteronomy 31:6)*

(continues)

- "I serve an awesome God who proclaims that He is my healer." *(Exodus 15:26)*
- "I am made in God's image and He has given my body the ability to heal itself." *(Genesis 1:27)*
- "I know that God will perfect that which concerns me to the end." *(Psalm 138:8)*

5. *Don't look back.* Don't beat yourself up over past decisions. Coping with that regret is key to maintaining proper physical and emotional health. Remind yourself that life is a journey, and we all make mistakes. Learn from them so you don't repeat them.

6. *Have a good cry by yourself.* Crying releases toxins from the body, including those found in cortisol, the stress hormone.[9] Crying is self-soothing and can actually improve your mood.[10]

7. *Cry with someone you trust.* Confide in a nonjudgmental friend, a loved one, or even a professional counselor who can relate to your situation. "Strong social and emotional support is a powerful stress buster that improves health and prolongs life," according to the American Institute of Stress.[11]

8. *Have faith.* Ask yourself, "Do I deserve to be well? Do I believe emotional balance and the abundant life are possible?" If your honest answer is yes, you're ready to move on. It's your God-given right to be happy, healthy, and emotionally stable. If your answer is no, you most likely have some forgiveness work to do and need to repeat points #1 and #2.

9. *Find a retreat.* A quiet, relaxing place in which to reflect is vital to restoring mental and emotional balance and finding your center. Visit a local park, take a walk or hike, or just find a place to sit and take in all God has created. Your health depends on it.

10. *Remove distractions.* While cleansing negative emotions, you are more susceptible to hurt. Be honest with yourself when opening

up to others and avoid people who feed on negative thoughts, as well as places associated with unpleasant memories.

11. *Ditch social media.* Take a break from Facebook and comparable sites, at least while you're in recovery. They can trigger feelings of jealousy and envy and cause you to develop unrealistic comparisons and even lead to depression.[12]

12. *Pamper yourself.* Regularly reward yourself with a nice long bath, a spa day, an aromatherapy session, or something else just for you. Also take time to pray or meditate. Individuals who live a spiritual life typically have better mental health and adapt more quickly to health problems than those who do not.[13]

Mental Abundance

A mind operating at peak performance extends beyond what we commonly think of as intelligence or IQ. It is not just being intellectual; instead, you must increase your overall mental capacity to grow in life. Doing so will allow you to be able to handle more projects, assume larger responsibilities, and live out your true potential. No wonder "brain training games" are in such high demand. They have been shown to enhance memory, executive function, attention, and even motor speed.[14,15]

Although technically an organ, the brain performs very much like a muscle, also operating under the "use it or lose it" principle. How do you train and strengthen your "mental muscles" to increase your mental capacity?

- *First and foremost, quit your "stinkin' thinkin'."* Just because a thought comes to mind doesn't mean it is a good thought. Learn to separate your thinking from who you are. The key to mental health is to voraciously curate your thoughts. Pick the weeds out of your mind as you would weeds in your garden. If you think you're fat, if you think you're ugly, if you think you're unhealthy, if you think you're stupid, you will be. But if you believe the opposite, you will be attractive, healthy, and intelligent.

- *Do new things that are just outside your comfort zone,* perhaps pursuing a new hobby, making friends with people from a culture other than your own, or listening to a different type of music. Or find the most unpleasant task in your to-do list and tackle it first.

- *Use the opposite side of your brain.* If you're left-side dominant, try something related to visual processing or simultaneously processing ideas to build up the right brain. For example, read a novel, create art, or play an instrument. If you're right-side dominant, consider tackling a task or test that involves deductive reasoning or working with facts and figures to challenge this part of your brain. Brain teasers and crossword puzzles qualify.

Once you build up your "brain muscles," it's vital to stop trying to control things. Don't sweat the small (or even the big) stuff. Let go of the incessant urge to know, and simply trust and let God's Spirit lead you. The reason why Tony Robbins and other motivational speakers are so popular is because they help people see through the haze that obscures what really matters. Jesus, Paul, and the apostles all spoke about the need to manage what's in your head. Robbins and others frame it in a less biblical way, although the timeless truth remains unchanged.

Physical Abundance

Maintaining a strong, healthy body is essential. The Bible refers to the body as the temple of the Holy Spirit, which has been "bought with a price; therefore, glorify God in your body" *(1 Corinthians 6:20).* You have a moral responsibility to take care of that body. By having a purpose that satisfies only oneself, it is all too easy to fall short as we lose focus and motivation to continue. No wonder most diets and exercise regimens fail. However, the obligation to eat right and stay fit to honor God supersedes a "me-centered" focus, all the while benefiting you in tangible ways.

Dr. Z here. It's crucial that you not be a victim of your circumstances at work. We've already discussed how sitting is the new smoking: It's a silent killer. People who sit all day live a few years less than active people.[16] In fact, sitting time is responsible for 4 percent of all deaths globally.[17] Sitting also slows your metabolism and interferes with your ability to find your healthy weight. It can also cause mental and emotional turmoil, which could spiral into health and spiritual ruin. This is another example of how all seven forms of abundance are crucial and connected.

Whether you're a truck driver or secretary, there are ways to be more active. Look into sitting calisthenics or sitting yoga. Stand up and stretch or take a walk down the hall every hour or so. Take fresh air breaks and walk or jog around the building. Squeeze in an exercise class on your lunch break. On a conference call, stand up and do some squats and lunges while you're at it. If you look weird, so be it. For more ideas, see Mama Z's exercise suggestions in the fitness section (see page 289).

Be sure to eat healthy on the job. (See Eating Well When Eating Out on page 150.) In addition to all the other reasons to care for your body, you want to look your best and project health, strength, and purpose as you begin your journey toward more soul-satisfying work.

Dr. Z here. When I used to bring my green juice drink to work every morning, people thought I was crazy. But who did they go to when they felt sick? Me. You can lead by example among your coworkers. Maybe you can convince your company to purchase desks that adjust from a sitting to a standing position, offer a group exercise class at lunch time or after work, or serve more fresh food in the company cafeteria.

LEARNING FROM THE BLUE ZONES

Let's revisit the Blue Zones we discussed in chapter 3. As you'll recall, these are the five places—the island of Sardinia, Okinawa, Costa Rica's Nicoya Peninsula, the Greek island of Ikaria, and Loma Linda, California—where elders live with vim and vigor to record-setting ages. Their lifestyles dovetail with an abundant life.[18]

1. *Live a life of motion.* Regular and sustained movement, including walking and gardening, is integral to their lives, and it is the only proven way to prevent cognitive decline.[19] Lacking many modern conveniences, most of them do things "by hand," requiring them to stay active.

2. *Keep the right outlook.* Blue Zoners actually have distinct words to express a sense of purpose and destiny for their lives. Prayer and slowing down the pace of one's lifestyle have been shown to reverse the inflammatory responses that are responsible for most chronic disease.

3. *Eat wisely.* Each Blue Zone population eats a predominantly plant-based diet, although a few also eat a moderate amount of meat. Most importantly, they don't overeat and have strategies to stave off gluttony. Okinawa, for example, has a three-thousand-year-old adage credited to Confucius that Okinawans recite before their meals to remind them to stop eating when their stomach is 80 percent full.

4. *Esteem your elders.* In Sardinia, honoring the aged—instead of regarding them as a burden—not only increases life expectancy, but also has benefited Sardinian youth.

5. *Never retire.* In Okinawa, there is no word for "retirement." Instead, elders work in whatever capacity they can, providing purpose and a sense of accomplishment, until the end of their days.

6. *Worship God.* The members of every Blue Zone have a direct connection to a divine purpose in their lives. The sense of belonging to a faith-based community has been proven to be worth an extra four to fourteen years of life expectancy to the Seventh-Day Adventists of Loma Linda, California.

7. *Build lifelong relationships.* Isolation kills. One group of five Okinawan women—average age one hundred and two—have known each other for ninety-seven years! Like most Blue Zoners, Adventists spend most of their time with like-minded people, so they remain encouraged to keep the principles that have worked so well over time.

Follow these seven key principles and you'll begin to experience the Abundant Life in no time!

Social Abundance

We discussed the importance of strong, healthy social relationships as the one common denominator of all the happiest places on earth above. Social abundance means spending time with people who support your healthy ways of life. We are both fit, and our closest friends are equally health oriented. We call them our "Fit Fam." We play volleyball together, exercise together, and go out and have fun together. You're not going to find a sad, lonely person among us, and if one of our friends is currently overweight, he or she is on the road to recovery. That's not to say that everyone has six-pack abs or looks like a swimsuit model, but we are all committed to bettering ourselves while also supporting and encouraging one another.

Who are *your* friends and the people you spend time with at work? If they're going to fast-food restaurants during lunch and drinking beer all night, remember that you are the company you keep. Focus on spending time with the people whose lives you want to emulate. Health is a big component of that. If no one you know is health minded, then join a group—or start one. Our community has a health and fitness group that meets once a week to discuss such issues. Your church or synagogue or community center may already have one. There is no excuse not to just open up the door and walk in.

Spiritual Abundance

We've left the best for last! Fulfilling your purpose in life is found in realizing that you are a spiritual being, created by a God who loves you, and that you have a wonderful destiny to fulfill. Many people struggle in their search for spiritual abundance. You may be shaking your head and saying, "This isn't possible for me." You are not alone. But if we continually seek a greater being in every aspect of our lives, we will be fulfilled and satisfied.

Living your faith in daily life keeps your spiritual muscles well toned; otherwise, they atrophy. To walk the walk every day, help the less fortunate, don't hurt others with your acts or words, and eschew guilty pleasures. Finally, don't let pride get in the way of seeking God's direction and help. Does the pot tell the potter how to form it? Nope. And neither should we.

Dr. Z here. My relationship with Christ didn't just dramatically change my own life. I am both proud and humbled to say that I have personally and professionally positively influenced countless others. Among the many changes that resulted in my transformation, including the transformation of my health, was my new way of eating, which I have shared in these pages. My heartfelt desire is that you, too, can experience this spiritual cleansing. Now let's hear from my partner in life.

Mama Z here. When I first felt the presence of God as a living spirit, it was the beginning of taking full responsibility for my physical health.

Now I am well and blessed that I can give back, by sharing this knowledge with our family, our friends, our community, the members of our church, and now the readers of this book.

The key to my success was staying balanced. To do all the things I do demands that I clearly define what is good—and not good—for me. I set boundaries, immovable boundaries, because once you move one boundary, the whole foundation begins to fall apart. This is the case regarding your weight, your mental health, your financial health. I propose that you adopt a way of life using essential oils, natural therapies, nutrition, exercise, and other healthy, holistic modalities to bring about a life of abundance.

Back to Your "Why"

We want to revisit a question we asked you earlier: "What is your *why*?" Why have you embarked on this journey of discovery and transformation?

Once you get past the immediate (but still compelling) objective of looking great in a bikini or getting your blood sugar down to a healthy level, what is your deeper motivation for following the Essential Oils Diet? What is it that will keep you following this new path?

In our experience, it is devotion to a higher power or a commitment to a larger purpose, followed by the desire to be of the greatest help to your family as possible, and lastly but importantly, to be healthy and look good. With all three of these reasons, how can you do anything but succeed in helping yourself—and others?

Quite simply, you can't have a robust spiritual life if you're an emotional wreck. Your emotions won't allow you to enjoy the spiritual abundance you might otherwise have. Whatever you're battling, there is hope. Your body has been designed by God to heal itself under the right conditions.

This book has given you the road map to those positive conditions. If you are still in doubt, go back and reread it. Know that if you do your part, God will do his part. Also realize, though, that you have free will. There's the law of reaping and sowing: If you sow a fast-food lifestyle, you will reap a fast-food body. But if you sow a healthy lifestyle, you'll reap what we Christians call biblical health, including a healthy body. The power of positive thinking, the power of prayer, and positive affirmations bring healing and health.

If there is one thing we have learned in life, it is to be patient with yourself. Don't get overwhelmed with a mountain of to-dos. Take each day as it comes. Celebrate successes—no matter how small or seemingly insignificant they may be—and give yourself a little grace.

We gradually add on responsibility—and accountability—to our children, and we should do the same for ourselves. Be patient. God's timing is not always on our timeline, and you may have to wait a while to get the answers you seek. Our hope and prayer is that you experience the abundant life in every area.

TIME FOR A REALITY CHECK

It is our fervent hope that you have experienced many transformational moments over the last thirty or more days. Likely you have lost some or all of the pounds to which you wanted to bid goodbye. Weight loss is hard to miss, but what if you have not made as much progress as you had hoped for, or are not sure if you've made as much progress in other areas? Are you uncertain about whether your health is in a better place now that you've been following the Essential Oils Diet? Whether it's your new way of eating or your new exercise regimen or any other new things you are doing to improve your health, it's crucial to get out your Transformation Journal and record the details of where you are now in comparison to where you were on Day 1.

First, go back and review your notes before you started the Essential Oils Diet. Be totally straight with yourself as you answer the following questions and set your new goals. Only you need ever see this! This is your journey, your body, your transformation.

- How do you feel overall? Are symptoms such as pain, brain fog, fatigue, and stress still nagging you?
- Are you experiencing transformation in any other areas of your life? How are your relationships going? Has your mood improved?
- How many pounds have you lost? Are you comfortable with the weight you have achieved? Do you feel that it is a healthy weight for your build and your age?
- Are your clothes fitting better? Sometimes you'll notice that before you see a difference on the scale—especially if you are more active than you were earlier. Or do you need to buy some new clothes because your pants are too loose?

- Has your energy level changed? Are you sleeping better? How's your love life?
- Are you enjoying the food you have been eating? Are you missing the foods you used to eat and have omitted?
- As you are in the process of transforming your body, what other habits have you changed? What else would you like to change in your life? Do you envision other transformations, whether in your relationships, your work, your spiritual practices, or any other aspect of your life?

Continue to review and make new entries in your journal. Tracking your progress as you journey along the road toward your goal weight and overall health is fundamental to staying accountable to your goals and remaining motivated to stay the course. And this is especially true when "life happens," as it inevitably does, or when you go through a rough period. Remember, you can always reread this book or zero in on a particular chapter to get yourself back on track.

Now turn to Part 3, where you'll find everything you need to follow the Essential Oils Diet, including recipes for easy-to-make and delectable dishes full of bioactive compounds and essential oils to feed body and soul. Most recipes are appropriate for both the Fast Track phase and Essential Lifestyle, aka the rest of your healthy life. The few that are suitable only for the latter are indicated as such with an asterisk in the Recipe Index on page 210. You'll also get a glimpse into Mama Z's kitchen and pantry with suggestions for ingredients and tools, as well as sources for products to replace the ones you will be eliminating.

Another twenty-six recipes for topical, oral, or inhaled aromatherapies will help speed weight loss, improve sleep, and boost energy, among other enhancements. They include appetite-control inhalers, massage oils, and tummy wraps to erase fat—and that's just for starters.

Our Essential Exercise section includes a series of moves to help you slim and tone your body as part of your overall commitment to becoming a body in motion. With these tools, you can build your personal program that suits you now and modify it as you continue your journey to permanent slimness, strength, and fitness.

PART 3

THE ESSENTIAL OILS DIET RECIPES, REMEDIES, AND EXERCISES

THE ESSENTIAL OILS DIET RECIPES

*M*ama Z here. We know that you are eager to get to our easy, slimming recipes full of bioactive compounds and tantalizing flavors. Many of these dishes are also enhanced by essential oils! All our recipes (or a variation) are suitable for vegetarians or vegans, and we also provide options in ingredients to suit most dietary restrictions. We have mastered the art of allergy-friendly cooking and want to help you have your (gluten-free, lactose-free, naturally sweetened) cake and eat it, too!

Cooking without processed sugar, wheat and other sources of gluten, and conventional dairy is easy once you get the hang of it. But if you are new to it, our list of alternative ingredients should be a big help. This is hardly an exhaustive list—the number of such products seems to grow daily. Most are available at Thrive Market, Whole Foods, your local health food store, and increasingly at well-stocked supermarkets. It would be a good idea to stock up before you begin the Essential Oils Diet.

Mama Z's Kitchen Makeover

This is what we have in our pantry at all times:

- All-purpose gluten-free flour, such as Trader Joe's or Bob's Red Mill (1-to-1 Baking Flour)
- Almond butter, such as Justin's non-GMO
- Almond flour, such as Bob's Red Mill
- Apple cider vinegar, such as Bragg Organic Raw Unfiltered
- Aluminum-free baking powder, such as Rumford
- Baking soda, such as Bob's Red Mill
- Bragg Liquid Aminos, a great replacement for soy sauce and Worcestershire sauce
- Bulletproof Coffee, made from organic beans specially roasted to minimize the formation of mold toxins
- Cacao powder, such as raw, organic GMO-free Natierra or TerrAmazon
- Chia seeds, such as Nutiva organic
- Coconut flour, such as Bob's Red Mill organic
- Canned (full-fat) coconut milk, such as Native Forest, organic and unsweetened
- Coconut sugar (aka coconut crystals), such as Nutiva organic
- DeBoles and Taste Republic gluten-free lasagna noodles and Cappello's gluten-free almond flour lasagna noodles
- Egg replacer, such as Namaste
- Chocolate chips, such as Enjoy Life mini chips, which are dairy-, gluten-, and soy-free; or Lily's dark chocolate chips, which are stevia sweetened without added sugar, vegan, and non-GMO
- Coconut oil, such as Carrington Farms raw, cold-pressed virgin, and organic
- Flax meal, such as Bob's Red Mill organic
- Whole flaxseed, such as Spectrum Essentials organic
- Ghee (organic and from grass-fed cows), such as Pure Traditions

- Gluten-free quick-cooking oats, such as Bob's Red Mill
- Grade A Dark or C maple syrup, such as Coombs Family Farms organic
- Maple sugar, such as Coombs Family Farms organic
- Living Fuel whole meal superfood (Greens, Berry, and Plant-Based Protein)
- Pasta Joy and Taste Republic gluten-free brown rice pastas and Cappello's gluten-free almond flour pastas
- Stevia (liquid) organic sweetener, such as SweetLeaf or KAL Sure Stevia, unflavored and flavored with vanilla, almond, coconut, lemon, and more
- Stevia (powdered) organic sweetener, such as KAL Sure Stevia extract powder
- Manuka (raw) honey, such as Wedderspoon or Manuka Health
- Mayonnaise made with avocado oil or grapeseed oil, such as Primal Kitchen or Follow Your Heart grapeseed or avocado oil vegenaise
- Pink Himalayan salt, such as Natierra Himalania
- Psyllium husk fiber, such as Yerba Prima
- Salmon, wild caught, such as Wild Planet non-GMO (canned) or Safe Catch wild tuna (pouch)
- Taco shells, such as Garden of Eden, organic
- Ujido matcha green tea powder
- Vegetable bouillon (organic), such as Rapunzel, which contains no hydrogenated oils
- Vanilla bean (organic) powder, such as Sunny Day Naturals

MAMA Z TIP

I always have a supply of mason jars in various sizes to store pantry items.

Now let's visit the fridge. Depending on your food sensitivities, you should find this list very helpful, especially if you're vegetarian, vegan, or simply want to minimize your intake of dairy and preservatives.

MAMA Z'S REFRIGERATOR AND FREEZER MAKEOVER

Instead of:	Use:
Bacon	Nitrate-free organic turkey bacon
Butter	Organic butter, preferably from grass-fed cows, or raw coconut oil
Cheese	Daiya, Kite Hill, So Delicious, Violife Foods, and Follow Your Heart dairy-free substitutes, or raw milk cheese (cow, goat, or sheep)
Condiments	Organicville agave-sweetened ketchup and Annie's mustard
Cream	Full-fat unsweetened canned organic coconut milk or coconut creamer
Cream cheese	Daiya and Kite Hill dairy-free substitutes
Deli meat	Applegate Farms organic sliced meats
Eggs	Local, organic, free-range eggs or egg replacer
Egg whites	Simple Truth Organic, 100% free-range eggs
Fresh pasta	Cappello's (gluten-free almond flour pasta) or Taste Republic gluten-free lasagna sheets, Miracle Noodle angel hair pasta and fettuccine (made with konjac flour)
Freezer meals	Carla Lee's nut tacos
Freezer meals (for kids)	Applegate Farms organic and gluten-free chicken nuggets and uncured beef corn dogs
Freezer meals (pizza)	Daiya, gluten-free
Ground meat	100% grass-fed beef; local is best
Half-and-half	Unsweetened Nutpods or Califia Farms Better Half "creamers"

Ice cream	So Delicious coconut milk ice cream (only the sugar-free variety; note that flavors other than vanilla may contain processed sugar, making them unacceptable)
Jams and jellies	BioNaturae All-Fruit Spread
Mayonnaise	Follow Your Heart grapeseed oil vegenaise or Primal Kitchen avocado oil mayo
Milk (whole)	Unsweetened and unsweetened vanilla almond milk or organic coconut milk
Ricotta cheese	So Delicious unsweetened coconut milk yogurt
Salad dressing	Homemade (see Recipe Index for our favorites)
Sour cream	Follow Your Heart grapeseed oil vegenaise
Yogurt	Unsweetened and unsweetened vanilla coconut milk yogurt

Other Important Substitutions

When you adapt your own recipes to our healthy way of eating, these tips should come in handy:

- If your recipe calls for 1 teaspoon vanilla extract and you're using an alternative sweetener (such as honey, honey crystals, coconut sugar, or stevia), increase the vanilla to 1 tablespoon.
- If a sweet recipe doesn't call for vanilla extract and you're using an alternative sweetener, add 1 teaspoon vanilla.
- A tablespoon of fresh herbs is the equivalent of 1 teaspoon of dried herbs.
- A tablespoon of fresh herbs, spices, citrus zest, and mint is the equivalent of two drops of essential oils.

Recipe Index

Recipes that are not suitable for the Fast Track phase of the Essential Diet have an asterisk (*) following the recipe name.

APPETIZERS

DINNERS

Recipe Key

The recipes that follow don't provide any nutritional facts. Why? Because they simply don't matter. The Essential Oils Diet doesn't require you to count calories or grams of carbs or fat. What a relief!

- Recipes that are *not* suitable for the Fast Track phase of the Essential Diet have an asterisk (*) following the recipe name. You can revisit these when you enter the Essential Lifestyle phase.
- Ingredients that are *not* suitable for the Fast Track phase also have an asterisk (*) following the ingredient. In most cases, there is another ingredient listed that can be substituted, making the recipe Fast Track–compliant.
- Sometimes a Note following a recipe provides more detail on less familiar ingredients. Many of them also appear on the pantry and refrigerator lists on pages 206 and 208.
- Organic foods are always preferable, as are fresh herbs.

A Note About Organic Ingredients

As we have made clear throughout this book, organically grown produce and other foods are the healthiest choices for you—and the environment. Organic produce and other ingredients are implicit in the following recipes. That being said, we realize that budget and availability may mean that it is not always possible to buy only organic products. For those reasons, and in the interest of space, we have *not* used the word *organic* before each ingredient in the following recipes. Let us also remind you to refer back to the Dirty Dozen (page 184) and the Clean Fifteen (page 185) for advice on which fresh fruits and vegetables are most likely to be sprayed with pesticides and therefore most important to buy organic, and which are least likely to be contaminated, meaning you may feel more comfortable buying them as conventionally grown produce.

For more specifics on recommended ingredients, see Mama Z's Kitchen Makeover on page 206.

For more specifics on recommended ingredients, see Mama Z's Kitchen Makeover on page 206.

BEVERAGES

Hibiscus-Green Iced Tea

To watch Mama Z make this refreshing green
tea, visit EssentialOilsDiet.com.

PREP: 5 MINUTES   STAND: 10 MINUTES   SERVES 4

2 green tea bags

2 hibiscus tea bags (coconut hibiscus, strawberry hibiscus, plain, or a mix)

4 dropperfuls liquid stevia

8 ounces boiling purified or distilled water

16 ounces cold purified or distilled water

Ice cubes

Place the green tea and hibiscus tea bags and the stevia in a 32-ounce glass water bottle. Add the boiling water. Steep for 10 minutes. Add the cold water and fill the bottle with ice.

Serve immediately or refrigerate.

Iced Matcha

PREP: 5 MINUTES   SERVES 2

1 tablespoon matcha green tea powder

2 cups unsweetened vanilla-flavored almond or coconut milk beverage, chilled, or unsweetened almond or coconut "creamer" (see Note, page 216)

4 dropperfuls vanilla- or coconut-flavored liquid stevia

Ice cubes

Pour the matcha powder, almond milk beverage, and stevia into a blender. Blend for 30 seconds, until frothy.

Pour the mixture into a 32-ounce glass bottle. Fill to the top with ice. Serve immediately or refrigerate.

Fat-Burning Iced Matcha

Add 2 drops each of cinnamon bark and peppermint essential oils.

Fat-Burning Matcha Latte

PREP: 5 MINUTES   SERVES 2

1 tablespoon matcha green tea powder

2 cups unsweetened vanilla-flavored almond or coconut milk beverage, heated, or unsweetened almond or coconut "creamer" (see Note, page 216)

2 cups boiling purified or distilled water

4 dropperfuls vanilla- or coconut-flavored liquid stevia

2 drops cinnamon bark essential oil

2 drops peppermint essential oil

1/2 teaspoon ground Ceylon cinnamon, plus more (optional) for garnish

Pour the matcha powder, almond milk, boiling water, stevia, essential oils, and cinnamon into a blender. Blend for 30 seconds, until frothy.

Pour into two 16-ounce glasses. Sprinkle more cinnamon on top, if desired. Serve immediately.

Nutpods and Califia Farms Better Half are both dairy-free half-and-half "creamers." Be sure to use an unsweetened variety.

Immune-Boosting Matcha Latte

Add 2 drops of our Immune-Boosting Blend to the latte. To make the blend, place 10 drops each of cinnamon bark, clove, eucalyptus, lemon, orange, and rosemary essential oils in a 5-ml bottle. Gently shake to combine.

Pumpkin-Spiced Matcha Latte

Add 1 drop each of cinnamon leaf, clove, and ginger essential oils to the Fat-Burning Matcha Latte.

Yerba Mate Iced Tea

PREP: 5 MINUTES   STAND: 10 MINUTES   SERVES 4

3 yerba mate tea bags

4 dropperfuls liquid stevia

8 ounces boiling purified or distilled water

16 ounces cold purified or distilled water

Ice cubes

Place the yerba mate and stevia in a 32-ounce glass water bottle. Add the boiling purified water. Steep for 10 minutes. Add the cold purified water to the bottle and fill to the top with ice.

Serve immediately or refrigerate.

Essential Water Concentrate

PREP: 5 MINUTES   SERVES 8

1 dropperful plain or flavored liquid stevia

10 drops lemon or lime essential oil

10 drops grapefruit or orange essential oil

1 tablespoon apple cider vinegar

1 teaspoon freshly squeezed lemon or lime juice

Purified or distilled water

1 scoop or packet electrolyte powder (optional; see Notes)

Put the liquid stevia and the essential oils, apple cider vinegar, and lemon juice into a 1-gallon glass water jug (see Notes). Fill to the top with purified water.

To make one serving, add 16 ounces of the concentrate into a 32-ounce glass container and fill with purified water.

For an added nutrition boost, add 1 scoop or packet of electrolyte powder and shake vigorously.

This is a four-day supply. Drink no more than 64 ounces each day because otherwise you'll exceed the maximum oral dose of essential oils as outlined in aromatherapy safety texts.

NOTES

We use Ultima electrolyte powder.

Large glass water jugs are available at many health food stores and at Whole Foods.

Heart-Healthy Blueberry Pancakes

PREP: 10 TO 15 MINUTES   COOK: 15 MINUTES   SERVES 6

3 large eggs, beaten

3 cups unsweetened vanilla-flavored almond milk beverage

2 cups gluten-free all-purpose flour* (use almond flour during Fast Track)

1/3 cup coconut flour

1/2 cup pecans or walnuts (or 1/4 cup of each)

1/2 cup almonds

1/4 cup flaxseeds

1 dropperful liquid stevia

1 tablespoon pure vanilla extract

1 teaspoon freshly ground pink Himalayan salt or sea salt

1 teaspoon aluminum-free baking powder

1 teaspoon baking soda

1 pint fresh blueberries, washed

1/4 cup unsweetened coconut flakes (optional)

2 tablespoons chia seeds (optional)

Olive-oil or coconut-oil cooking spray

Put the eggs and almond milk in a blender or food processor and give them a quick pulse. Add the flours, pecans, almonds, flaxseeds, stevia, vanilla, and Himalayan salt, and blend until the mixture is completely smooth. Add the baking powder and baking soda.

Transfer the mixture to a large measuring cup or a medium bowl with a spout. Stir in the blueberries and, if desired, the coconut flakes and chia seeds.

Heat a griddle or flat pan over medium heat and mist it with the cooking spray. Using a spoon, drip a few test drops of batter on the griddle. Once they puff up and brown nicely, ladle 1/4 to 1/3 cup batter for each pancake onto the griddle. When little bubbles on top of the batter pop and stay popped, flip the pancakes. You will probably need to mist the griddle again with the cooking spray between batches. Place the cooked pancakes on a plate and put in a warm oven until all are done.

Serve with maple syrup or fresh berries if desired.

Make the batter the night before and put it in the fridge, covered, until morning. If it firms up, add a little more almond milk beverage to get the right consistency.

Heart-Healthy Blueberry Waffles

Use the same recipe and follow manufacturer's instructions for the waffle iron. You may have to mist the waffle iron with cooking spray between batches.

Mama Z's Super Greens Powder

This recipe is not for everybody. It makes enough for a year. The same goes for the recipe for Super Reds (page 221). You cannot buy most of these ingredients in quantities of less than a pound or without paying significantly more per ounce for smaller quantities. If you are unable to buy in bulk or do not want to use it daily, consider purchasing Living Fuel SuperGreens and/or SuperBerry (page 104) instead.

PREP: 30 MINUTES   MAKES 365 SERVINGS

1 pound bee pollen powder

1 pound unsweetened cacao powder

1 pound chia seeds

1 pound chlorella powder

1 pound ginkgo leaf powder

1 pound gotu kola powder

1 pound guarana powder

1 pound hemp protein powder

1 pound kelp powder

1 pound red maca powder

8 ounces noni powder

1 pound pumpkinseed powder

1 pound spirulina powder

4 ounces stevia powder

4 ounces raw VitaCherry powder

1 pound ground cinnamon

1 pound ground ginger

Place the bee pollen, cacao, chia seeds, chlorella, ginkgo leaf, gotu kola, guarana, hemp protein, kelp, red maca, noni, pumpkinseed, spirulina, stevia, and VitaCherry powders, and the ground cinnamon and ginger in a large cooler or other container. Stir with a large wire whisk or slotted spoon until the ingredients are completely mixed.

Divide the mixture into fifteen 1-pound packages and store in food-grade plastic or glass containers away from sunlight and heat.

Use 2 tablespoons in each Mama Z's Bioactive Breakfast Shake (page 222) or other 15-ounce shake.

MAMA Z TIP

I buy all these ingredients from Nuts.com or Amazon.com. The recipe makes enough for a year for one person, which comes to about $9 to $10 a month, significantly less than purchasing a commercial greens powder. I try to get organic and raw ingredients whenever possible. You might also want to go in with a friend or three and divide the packages among yourselves.

Mama Z's Super Reds Powder

PREP: 30 MINUTES   MAKES 365 SERVINGS

4 ounces acai powder

1 pound apple cider vinegar powder

4 ounces baobab fruit powder

1 pound beet powder

4 ounces raw wild blueberry powder

4 ounces camu camu powder

1 pound dandelion root powder

1 pound echinacea powder

1 pound fenugreek powder

8 ounces garcinia cambogia

8 ounces glucomannan powder

8 ounces goji berry powder

1 pound hawthorn berry powder

4 ounces mangosteen powder

4 ounces wild maqui powder

2 ounces monk fruit powder

1 pound mulberry leaf powder

8 ounces pomegranate powder

8 ounces strawberry powder

4 ounces raw VitaCherry powder

8 ounces vitamin C powder

8 ounces yacon powder

4 ounces yumberry powder

Place the acai, apple cider vinegar, baobab fruit, beet, wild blueberry, camu camu, dandelion root, echinacea, fenugreek, garcinia cambogia, glucomannan, goji berry, hawthorn berry, mangosteen, wild maqui, monk fruit, mulberry leaf, pomegranate, strawberry, VitaCherry, vitamin C, yacon, and yumberry powders in a large cooler or other container. Stir with a wire whisk or slotted spoon until completely mixed.

Divide into thirteen 1-pound packages and store in food-grade plastic or glass containers out of sunlight and heat.

Use 2 tablespoons in Mama Z's Bioactive Breakfast Shake (page 222) or other 15-ounce shake.

Mama Z's Bioactive Breakfast Shake

PREP: 10 MINUTES   SERVES 1

4 to 6 ounces purified or distilled water

2 tablespoons Mama Z's Super Greens Powder (page 220) or Living Fuel SuperGreens

2 tablespoons Mama Z's Super Reds Powder (page 221) or Living Fuel SuperBerry

2 tablespoons vegan brown rice protein powder or Living Fuel LivingProtein

1/2 banana

1/4 cup frozen raspberries, blueberries, blackberries, pitted cherries, or other dark berries

Unsweetened vanilla-flavored almond or coconut milk beverage

Place the purified water, Mama Z's Super Greens and Super Reds powders, brown rice protein powder, banana, and frozen berries in a blender or Magic Bullet. Add the almond milk to bring the total to 16 ounces. Blend thoroughly and pour into a large glass.

MAMA Z TIP

You can also enjoy this nutritious shake as a meal replacement or a pick-me-up in the late afternoon.

Greens and Herb Omelet

PREP: 5 MINUTES   COOK: 10 MINUTES   SERVES 2

6 large eggs, or 1 (16-ounce) carton egg whites

2 tablespoons unsweetened almond or coconut milk beverage

2 drops basil, dill, or another herbal essential oil (optional)

2 tablespoons raw coconut oil, extra-virgin olive oil, or butter

Large handful of coarsely chopped vegetables, such as fresh or frozen spinach, kale, broccoli, or asparagus, or any combination

1/2 cup dairy-free Cheddar-style shredded cheese alternative or mozzarella-style shreds (see Note, page 228)

Pinch of freshly ground pink Himalayan salt or sea salt

Pinch of freshly ground white pepper

1/2 tablespoon chopped fresh basil, dill, or other herbs, or 1/2 teaspoon dried (optional)

If using whole eggs, beat them in a small bowl with the almond milk and essential oil, if using, until frothy and well blended. Alternatively, add the almond milk and the herbal essential oil, if using, to the egg-white container and shake.

Melt the coconut oil in a medium sauté pan over medium heat. Add the vegetables and sauté briefly, until slightly limp. Add the beaten egg–almond milk mixture to the pan, followed by the cheese alternative, Himalayan salt, white pepper, and chopped basil, if using.

When the mixture starts to firm up, gently flip it over and cook until the eggs are no longer runny when the pan is tilted, about 2 minutes. Cut the omelet in half, slide it onto two warm plates, and serve.

MAMA Z TIP

Double this recipe and, after cooking, refrigerate half of it in a covered glass container for up to three days. Reheat in a convection or traditional oven at 325°F for 15 to 20 minutes. Serve as breakfast another day or over a bed of organic greens for lunch.

Nutty Chocolate Protein Smoothie

PREP: 5 MINUTES   SERVES 1

1 frozen banana, peeled

1 tablespoon chia seeds

1 tablespoon flaxseeds

1 tablespoon raw cacao powder

1/2 Hass avocado, peeled and pitted

1/2 cup chopped fresh or frozen mango

Handful of almonds

1 serving (according to the product label) vegan protein powder, such as organic brown rice protein powder or Living Fuel LivingProtein

Unsweetened almond or coconut milk beverage

Ice cubes (optional)

Place the banana, chia seeds, flaxseeds, cacao powder, avocado, mango, almonds, and protein powder in a blender. Add almond milk to cover the other ingredients. Add ice cubes, if desired.

Blend until thoroughly mixed.

Berry Green Delight Smoothie

PREP: 5 MINUTES   SERVES 1

1 frozen banana, peeled

1 cup frozen mixed berries

1 cup torn fresh spinach or kale leaves

1/2 ripe Hass avocado, peeled and pitted

2 tablespoons Mama Z's Super Greens Powder (page 220) or Living Fuel SuperGreens

Unsweetened almond or coconut milk beverage

Ice cubes (optional)

Place the banana, berries, spinach, avocado, and greens powder in a blender. Add enough almond milk to cover the other ingredients. Add ice cubes, if desired.

Blend thoroughly and enjoy.

Cacao Energy Bowl

PREP: 5 MINUTES   SERVES 1

1 bag frozen acai berries (see Note)

1 frozen banana, peeled

1/2 Hass avocado, peeled and pitted

2 tablespoons Mama Z's Super Greens Powder (page 220) or Living Fuel SuperGreens

1 tablespoon raw cacao powder

1 teaspoon matcha green tea powder (see page 207)

Handful of chopped fresh kale

Handful of fresh or frozen spinach

1/2 to 1 cup unsweetened almond or coconut milk beverage

Fresh banana slices, for garnish

Unsweetened coconut flakes, for garnish

Hempseeds, for garnish

Chia seeds, for garnish

Place the acai berries, banana, avocado, greens powder, cacao powder, matcha powder, kale, and spinach in a blender. Add 1/2 cup almond milk and blend, using the tamping tool to ensure the ingredients are thoroughly mixed. Add more almond milk as needed to reach the desired consistency.

Pour the mixture into a bowl and garnish with banana slices, coconut flakes, hempseeds, and chia seeds.

NOTE
Most stores sell frozen acai berries in individual serving sizes of 100 grams.

Spicy Autumn Breakfast Bake*

PREP: 30 MINUTES   COOK: 50 TO 60 MINUTES   STAND: 15 MINUTES   SERVES 4

2 large eggs

1¹/2 cups leftover cooked gluten-free oats, quinoa, or brown rice

1 (13.5-ounce) can full-fat unsweetened coconut milk

1¹/2 cups unsweetened vanilla-flavored almond milk beverage

1 teaspoon pure vanilla extract

¹/4 cup coconut sugar, or 3 dropperfuls plain liquid stevia

¹/2 cup raisins or other chopped dried fruit

¹/2 teaspoon freshly ground pink Himalayan salt or sea salt

¹/2 tablespoon pumpkin pie spice (see Note, page 260)

1 drop cinnamon essential oil

1 drop ginger essential oil

1 drop clove essential oil

1 drop nutmeg essential oil

Preheat the oven to 325°F.

In an ungreased 1¹/2-quart casserole dish, beat the eggs until fluffy. Stir in the leftover oats, coconut milk, almond milk, vanilla, coconut sugar, raisins, Himalayan salt, pumpkin pie spice, and the essential oils, mixing well.

Bake uncovered for 50 to 60 minutes, stirring every 15 minutes, until most of the liquid is absorbed. Remove from the oven. The top of the porridge may be wet and not fully set. Be careful not to overbake or it may curdle.

Stir well and let the porridge stand for at least 15 minutes. The more time it has to settle and cool, the more the liquid will be absorbed. (For ultimate creamy goodness, place it in the refrigerator overnight.) Serve cold or reheat in a 325°F oven for 15 to 30 minutes.

Quick Tuna or Salmon Salad

PREP: 15 MINUTES   SERVES 1

1 (5- to 7-ounce) can or vacuum-packed pouch of wild tuna or pink salmon, drained

2 tablespoons grapeseed-oil or avocado-oil vegan mayonnaise

1 teaspoon Dijon or yellow mustard

1 teaspoon dill pickle relish, or 1 small dill pickle, chopped

1 stalk celery, chopped

1 drop dill essential oil

1/3 cup halved grapes, whole blueberries, or chopped apple

1/4 teaspoon freshly ground Pink Himalayan salt or sea salt

1/8 teaspoon freshly ground white pepper

3 small cooked beets, cut into 1/2-inch pieces

1/4 cup chopped pecans or walnuts (optional)

2 cups chopped greens

In a medium bowl, combine the tuna, vegan mayonnaise, mustard, relish, celery, dill essential oil, grapes, Himalayan salt, white pepper, beets, and pecans (if using), and gently mix.

Serve over the greens.

Avocado Egg Salad

PREP: 20 MINUTES   SERVES 1

3 large eggs

1 tablespoon grapeseed-oil or avocado-oil vegan mayonnaise

1 teaspoon Dijon mustard

1 stalk celery, chopped

1/8 teaspoon dried dill

1/8 teaspoon paprika

1 drop dill essential oil

1/4 teaspoon freshly ground Pink Himalayan salt or sea salt

1/8 teaspoon freshly ground white pepper

1/2 medium Hass avocado, peeled, pitted, and cut into 1/2-inch pieces

1/4 cup chopped pecans or walnuts (optional)

Place the eggs in a small saucepan and cover with water. Bring the water to a boil over high heat, then immediately turn off the heat. Cover the saucepan and let it sit for 15 minutes. Drain the hot water and run cold water over the eggs for a minute or two. Shell and halve the eggs, then cut them up and place in a bowl.

Add the vegan mayonnaise, mustard, celery, dill, paprika, dill essential oil, Himalayan salt, white pepper, avocado, and, if desired, pecans. Stir to blend. Serve plain or on a bed of greens. The egg salad may be refrigerated, covered, for up to three days.

MAMA Z TIP

To make fast work of cutting up hard-boiled eggs, use an egg or strawberry cutting tool. Cut one way and then switch directions. I can cut three eggs in less than a minute this way.

Super Greens and Cucumber Salad

PREP: 10 MINUTES   SERVES 4 TO 6

APPLE CIDER VINAIGRETTE

1 cup extra-virgin olive oil

1/4 cup apple cider vinegar

1 large egg, or 1 tablespoon egg replacer plus 2 tablespoons purified or distilled water

1 teaspoon chopped fresh chives

1 teaspoon dried Italian herb blend or herbes de Provence

1/2 teaspoon freshly ground pink Himalayan salt or sea salt

1/4 teaspoon freshly ground white pepper

SALAD

2 cups finely chopped bok choy stalks and leaves

2 cups Tuscan kale or other kale (first remove stem and spine and then tear into small pieces)

2 cups baby spinach

2 large cucumbers, peeled, seeded, and thinly sliced

Chia sprouts or your favorite sprouts or microgreens, for garnish

For the apple cider vinaigrette: Pour the olive oil into a mini blender or whisk it in a bowl. Slowly pour in the cider vinegar to emulsify. Add the egg and blend thoroughly. Season with the chives, dried herbs, Himalayan salt, and white pepper. Set aside while you make the salad.

For the salad: Toss the bok choy, kale, spinach, and cucumbers in a salad bowl. As you plate the salad, top each serving with a small amount of chia sprouts. Drizzle with the vinaigrette.

Super Greens Summer Salad

PREP: 15 MINUTES   SERVES 2 TO 4

5 cups cubed watermelon

1 pint blueberries

Juice of ½ lemon

1 dropperful liquid stevia

2 tablespoons finely chopped fresh mint

½ cup vegan dairy-free feta alternative or vegan mozzarella-style shreds (optional; see Note)

2 cups baby spinach

2 cups Tuscan kale or other kale (remove stem and spine and tear into small pieces before measuring)

Pinch of freshly ground pink Himalayan salt or sea salt

In a large bowl, combine the cubed watermelon and blueberries. Pour the lemon juice and stevia over the top. Sprinkle on the mint and the vegan cheese, if using. Toss thoroughly to combine.

Toss the spinach and kale together in a large bowl. Top with the fruit and cheese mixture. Sprinkle with Himalayan salt.

NOTE
Good brands of dairy-free cheese include Kite Hill, Daiya, So Delicious, Violife Foods, and Follow Your Heart.

Essentially Delicious Yogurt

PREP: 5 MINUTES   SERVES 4 OR 5

1 (24-ounce) container unsweetened vanilla coconut- or almond-milk yogurt alternative

1 drop lemon, orange, lime, or grapefruit essential oil

4 dropperfuls plain or vanilla-flavored liquid stevia

$^1/_3$ cup dried, dehydrated, or freeze-dried fruit pieces (without added sugar or other ingredients)

$^1/_2$ cup raw sliced or slivered almonds (optional)

$^1/_4$ cup chia seeds (optional)

$^1/_4$ cup hempseeds (optional)

Using an immersion blender, a blender, or a food processor, mix together the yogurt alternative, essential oil, stevia, and dried fruit.

Ladle the mixture evenly into cups or parfait glasses. Top with the almonds, chia seeds, and/or hempseeds, if desired.

MAMA Z TIP

This recipe is amazingly versatile and a real kid favorite (halve the portions for younger kids). Use vanilla-flavored liquid stevia with unsweetened yogurt substitute or plain liquid stevia for unsweetened vanilla yogurt substitute, unless you like extra vanilla flavor as we do. Instead of dried fruit, you can use $^1/_3$ cup powdered strawberry, raspberry, blueberry, mango, pineapple, or apple. Or try $^1/_4$ cup raw cacao powder in lieu of fruit.

Mama Z's Coleslaw

To watch Mama Z make this cruciferous
coleslaw, visit EssentialOilsDiet.com.

PREP: 10 MINUTES   CHILL: 6 HOURS   SERVES 8

SLAW

1 (12-ounce) bag broccoli slaw or kale
slaw, 1 small head cabbage, or 1 or 2
finely shredded large carrots and the
finely shredded stalks from a head of
broccoli (about 2 cups)

1/4 cup raisins or currants

1/4 cup chopped walnuts

1 cup peeled, cored, and chopped
apple (1 large apple)

DRESSING

2/3 cup grapeseed-oil or avocado-oil
vegan mayonnaise

3 tablespoons apple cider vinegar

1 dropperful plain liquid stevia

1 drop coriander essential oil

2 tablespoons unsweetened almond
milk beverage

Dash of freshly ground pink Himalayan
salt or sea salt

Dash of freshly ground white pepper

For the slaw: In a medium mixing bowl, combine the shredded vegetables, raisins, walnuts, and apple.

For the dressing: In a blender or Magic Bullet, combine the vegan mayonnaise,
cider vinegar, liquid stevia, coriander essential oil, almond milk, Himalayan salt,
and white pepper, and blend.

Pour the dressing over the slaw and toss to mix thoroughly. Serve immediately
or refrigerate, covered, for up to 6 hours.

Spiced Butternut Squash Soufflé*

PREP: 15 MINUTES   COOK: 1 HOUR   SERVES 6 TO 8

½ cup butter or raw coconut oil, melted, plus more for greasing

2 cups cooked and mashed butternut squash

1 teaspoon freshly ground pink Himalayan salt or sea salt

5 to 6 tablespoons Grade A Dark or C maple syrup, or 5 to 6 dropperfuls plain liquid stevia

3 tablespoons non-GMO cornstarch

3 large eggs

1¼ cups unsweetened canned full-fat coconut milk

2 drops cinnamon essential oil

1 drop ginger essential oil

2 drops clove essential oil

2 drops nutmeg essential oil

½ cup slivered or sliced almonds

Preheat the oven to 350°F. Grease a 1½-quart casserole.

Combine the squash, salt, maple syrup, and cornstarch in a food processor or large blender (see Note). Blend until fluffy. Add the eggs, coconut milk, and butter, and mix thoroughly. Drop the essential oils through the chute in the food processor or hole in the blender top and combine.

Pour the mixture into the prepared casserole. Sprinkle with the almonds. Bake for 1 hour or until a toothpick inserted in the center comes out clean.

Serve hot.

NOTE
If you don't have a blender or food processor, separate the eggs and beat the whites until fluffy before gently folding them into the squash mixture.

Basil, Garlic, and Pine Nut Super Pasta

PREP: 30 MINUTES   COOK: 5 MINUTES   SERVES 4

4 medium garlic cloves, minced

3 tablespoons extra-virgin olive oil, plus more as needed

1 teaspoon freshly ground Pink Himalayan salt or sea salt, plus more for the pot

1 (9-ounce) package brown rice fettuccine or linguine pasta* (use frozen almond flour or Miracle Noodle fettuccine while on Fast Track)

1/2 teaspoon freshly ground white pepper

1/2 cup lightly toasted pine nuts

1 cup vegan mozzarella- or Parmesan-style shreds (see Note, page 233)

10 to 12 large basil leaves, shredded

Fill a large pot with water and bring it to a boil over high heat.

Meanwhile, in a large sauté pan over low heat, soften the garlic in the olive oil. Remove the pan from the heat, cover, and set it aside to keep warm.

When the water boils, salt it well, add fresh pasta with a little olive oil, and cook, stirring it every few seconds, until it is al dente, about 3 minutes. If you're using dried pasta, follow the package directions, turning off the heat at the lower end of the cooking time and stir until you reach the higher number. (For example, if the package indicates 7 to 10 minutes, turn off the heat at 7 minutes and stir for 3 more minutes.) Drain the pasta, reserving 3/4 cup of the cooking water, rinse, and drain again. Add the drained pasta to the sauté pan with 1/2 cup of the reserved cooking water, 1 teaspoon Himalayan salt, and the white pepper.

In a serving bowl, toss the pasta with the pine nuts, 3/4 cup of the vegan cheese, and the shredded basil. The sauce should just coat the pasta. If desired, add a little more pasta water or drizzle it lightly with extra-virgin olive oil. Sprinkle with the remaining cheese substitute. Serve hot.

NOTE
Good brands of dairy-free cheese include Kite Hill, Daiya, So Delicious, Violife Foods, and Follow Your Heart.

VARIATIONS
Instead of almond or brown rice pasta, use well-rinsed and drained cooked Miracle Noodle fettuccine or linguine. Or omit the pasta altogether and instead toss with zoodles (spiralized zucchini, seeded if large) or fresh spinach, or serve over a spinach salad. (Zoodles can be boiled for 2 minutes or served raw.)

MAMA Z TIP

To toast pine nuts, place them in a small dry skillet and cook over medium-low heat, stirring constantly, until fragrant and lightly browned, 2 to 4 minutes.

Sweet Potato Falafel

PREP: 15 MINUTES   COOK: 40 TO 80 MINUTES   CHILL: 1 HOUR OR MORE
SERVES 4 TO 6

2 medium sweet potatoes (about 1¹/₂ pounds)

2 medium garlic cloves, pressed

1 teaspoon ground cumin

1 teaspoon ground coriander

1 small bunch cilantro, de-stemmed and chopped

Juice of ¹/₂ lemon

1 cup gluten-free all-purpose flour* (use almond flour while on Fast Track), plus more as needed

¹/₂ teaspoon freshly ground pink Himalayan salt or sea salt

¹/₄ teaspoon freshly ground white pepper

1 drop cumin essential oil

1 drop coriander essential oil

1 drop lemon essential oil

Olive-oil or coconut-oil cooking spray

Vegan mayonnaise

Steam the whole sweet potatoes for about 25 minutes in a steamer over simmering water until you can put a fork all the way through them. Alternatively, preheat the oven to 350°F, poke a few holes in each sweet potato, and bake for 45 to 60 minutes, until they are easily pierced with a fork. Allow the steamed or baked sweet potatoes to cool just enough to handle, then plunge them briefly into cold water and peel.

Using a stand mixer or food processor, blend the sweet potatoes, garlic, cumin, coriander, cilantro, lemon juice, almond flour, Himalayan salt, white pepper, and the essential oils until the mixture is smooth.

Place the mixture in the refrigerator for at least 1 hour to firm up. It should be sticky, but if it is too wet to work with, add 1 tablespoon of flour at a time until it is firm enough.

Preheat the oven to 400°F. Mist a baking sheet with the cooking spray.

Using a cookie scoop, large spoon, or small measuring cup, form ¹/₄ to ¹/₃ cup of dough at a time into a ball; you should have 20 balls. Place them on the prepared baking sheet, leaving space between them, and flatten them slightly with the tines of a fork. Bake for 15 to 20 minutes, until the patties are brown on top.

Remove from the oven and allow to set for 2 minutes. As they can be fragile, depending on the gluten-free flour used, carefully place them over a salad or greens on a serving dish or individual plates. Serve with vegan mayonnaise.

Tasty Tomato Bisque

PREP: 20 MINUTES   COOK: 20 MINUTES   SERVES 5 OR 6

3/4 cup chopped yellow onion, or 1/4 cup dried onion

1/2 cup butter or raw coconut oil

3/4 teaspoon dried dillseed

1 tablespoon chopped fresh dill, or 1 teaspoon dried

1 tablespoon chopped fresh oregano, or 1 teaspoon dried

1/4 cup gluten-free all-purpose flour* (use almond flour while on Fast Track)

3 to 4 cups fresh or canned diced tomatoes

3 cups vegetable stock

1 1/2 teaspoons freshly ground pink Himalayan salt or sea salt

1/2 teaspoon freshly ground white pepper

1/4 cup chopped fresh parsley

2 drops dill essential oil

2 drops oregano essential oil

2 drops lemon essential oil

1 1/4 cups raw honey* (use 1 dropperful liquid stevia while on Fast Track)

1 (13.5-ounce) can full-fat unsweetened coconut milk (1 1/2 cups)

In a medium saucepan over low heat, sauté the onions with the butter, dillseed, and chopped dill and oregano. Add the flour, stirring for 2 minutes. Gradually stir in the tomatoes, alternating with the vegetable stock. Add the Himalayan salt, white pepper, and parsley. Raise the heat to medium and bring to a gentle boil; reduce the heat and simmer for 15 minutes.

Add the essential oils, honey, and coconut milk. Using an immersion blender, mix well. Heat through and ladle the soup into bowls. Serve either hot or cold. Refrigerate any leftovers for up to four days.

Kale and Lentil Super Soup

PREP: 10 TO 15 MINUTES COOK: 45 MINUTES SERVES 4

1/4 cup extra-virgin olive oil

1 medium sweet Vidalia onion, finely chopped, or 2 tablespoons dried

4 medium garlic cloves, pressed

2 medium carrots, sliced

1 teaspoon ground cumin

1 teaspoon curry powder

1/4 teaspoon dried thyme

1 (28-ounce) can diced tomatoes, drained, or 28 ounces of tomato sauce

3 drops lemon essential oil

2 or 3 drops cumin essential oil

1 drop thyme essential oil

1 cup mixed red, green, and brown lentils, rinsed

4 cups vegetable broth

2 cups boiling purified or distilled water

1 tablespoon freshly squeezed lemon or lime juice

1 teaspoon freshly ground pink Himalayan salt or sea salt

1/2 teaspoon freshly ground white pepper

1/4 teaspoon cayenne pepper

2 small bunches baby kale, chopped, or 1 (10-ounce) bag frozen kale

Heat the olive oil in a large pot over medium heat. Add the onion, garlic, and carrots. Cook until the onion and garlic are very tender and starting to brown, about 10 minutes. Add the cumin, curry powder, and thyme, and cook, stirring, for 30 seconds to 1 minute to release their scent. Stir in the tomatoes, followed by the essential oils.

Pour in the lentils, broth, 1 cup of the boiling water, and the lemon juice. Add the Himalayan salt, white pepper, and cayenne. Bring the mixture to a boil over medium heat and immediately reduce the heat to low. Simmer for 20 to 30 minutes, until the lentils are cooked through and tender.

Using an immersion blender, puree the entire mixture. Then add the kale and the remaining 1 cup of boiling water. Cook for another 5 to 10 minutes over low heat, until the kale is cooked through.

If not serving immediately, refrigerate for up to five days or freeze the soup in smaller portions.

Sam's Bruschetta*

PREP: 10 TO 15 MINUTES   COOK: 3 TO 5 MINUTES   SERVES 8 TO 10

4 plum tomatoes, seeded and chopped

1/2 cup dairy-free mozzarella-style or Parmesan-style cheese shreds (see Note, page 233)

1/4 cup minced fresh basil

2 tablespoons minced fresh parsley

3 medium garlic cloves, minced

3 tablespoons extra-virgin olive oil

2 teaspoons balsamic vinegar

1 or 2 drops basil essential oil

1/8 teaspoon freshly ground pink Himalayan salt or sea salt

1/8 teaspoon crushed red pepper flakes

1/8 teaspoon freshly ground white pepper

2 (8.4-ounce) gluten-free baguettes, cut in 1/2-inch slices, or 6 dinner rolls (halved)

1/4 cup butter or raw coconut oil, softened

2 cups dairy-free mozzarella-style cheese shreds

Preheat the broiler to low.

In a small bowl, combine the tomatoes, the 1/2 cup mozzarella-style shreds, the basil, parsley, garlic, olive oil, balsamic vinegar, basil essential oil, Himalayan salt, red pepper flakes, and white pepper. Set aside.

Spread the baguette slices with the butter. Top each slice with some of the 2 cups mozzarella-style shreds.

Place the baguette slices on an ungreased baking sheet. Broil 3 to 4 inches from the heat for 3 to 5 minutes, until the cheese melts. Watch carefully to avoid burning the cheese or the bread. Remove from the oven.

With a slotted spoon, top each baguette slice with about 1 tablespoon of the tomato mixture (see Note). Place on a tray and serve.

NOTE
You will have some bread left over that you can toast lightly and toss in a food processor to make bread crumbs for other meals.

Lemon Dip with Essential Oils*

PREP: 10 MINUTES   CHILL: 8 HOURS   SERVES 8 (4 CUPS)

2 cups Natural Confectioners' Sugar (page 262)

1 cup unsweetened plain coconut milk yogurt alternative

1 (8-ounce) container dairy-free almond cream cheese or plain cream cheese-style spread (see Note, page 242)

1 teaspoon grated lemon zest

2 tablespoons freshly squeezed lemon juice

1 tablespoon dried lemon balm (see Note)

9 drops lemon essential oil, or 1 tablespoon pure lemon extract

4 dropperfuls lemon-flavored liquid stevia

Place the confectioners' sugar, yogurt alternative, dairy-free cream cheese, lemon zest, lemon juice, lemon balm, lemon essential oil, and stevia in a food processor or large blender and blend for 1 to 2 minutes, until thoroughly combined.

Transfer to a serving dish and refrigerate overnight to set. Serve with fruit and/ or gluten-free crackers or gluten-free pretzels.

NOTE
Dried lemon balm, or melissa, is the secret ingredient in this recipe. You'll find it in the herb section of health food stores or at Whole Foods.

Kale and Avocado Super Pesto

PREP: 15 MINUTES   SERVES 12 TO 20

1 ripe Hass avocado, peeled and pitted

10 ounces Tuscan or curly kale, spines and stems removed

2 3/4 cups fresh basil leaves

1 ounce fresh thyme, de-stemmed

8 medium garlic cloves

3/4 cup purified or distilled water

1/4 cup freshly squeezed lemon or lime juice

1 teaspoon freshly ground pink Himalayan salt or sea salt

1/2 teaspoon freshly ground white pepper

2 drops lemon or lime essential oil

In a food processor or blender, place the avocado, kale, basil, thyme, garlic, purified water, lemon juice, Himalayan salt, white pepper, and lemon essential oil. Pulse the mixture until well combined, then process continuously for 1 minute.

Scoop into a serving dish and serve with Marcona almonds or almond crackers. Refrigerate any leftovers in an airtight container for up to three days.

VARIATION: BROWN RICE VEGGIE WRAPS WITH PESTO
Fill brown rice or veggie wraps with salad and top with pesto. Alternatively, serve the pesto over a salad.

Sun-Dried Tomato Pesto

PREP: 10 TO 15 MINUTES   MAKES 2 CUPS

3/4 cup oil-packed sun-dried tomatoes

Extra-virgin olive oil

8 medium garlic cloves

1/4 cup pine nuts, silvered almonds, or Marcona almonds

1/4 cup snipped fresh basil, or 1 tablespoon dried, crushed

3 drops basil essential oil

1/2 teaspoon freshly ground pink Himalayan salt or sea salt

Drain the tomatoes, reserving the oil. Add enough olive oil to the drained oil to make 1/2 cup and set it aside.

Combine the drained tomatoes, garlic, pine nuts, basil, basil essential oil, and Himalayan salt in a food processor or blender. Cover and process until finely chopped.

With the machine running, gradually add the reserved oil, processing until almost smooth, stopping to scrape down the sides of the bowl as needed.

Serve with almond crackers or gluten-free pretzels. Divide any leftover pesto into small containers to freeze or refrigerate.

Pesto Cream "Cheese" Dip

Mix 1/3 cup pesto with one 8-ounce package dairy-free cream cheese-style spread or almond milk cream cheese. Puree all the ingredients in a food processor or blender for 1 to 2 minutes. Transfer to a serving bowl, cover and refrigerate at least 2 hours or up to overnight. Serve with raw vegetables or gluten-free chips.

VARIATION
Mix dairy-free cream cheese with Kale and Avocado Super Pesto (page 238) or Basil and Parsley Super Pesto (page 240).

Basil and Parsley Super Pesto

PREP: 10 TO 15 MINUTES   MAKES 2¹/₂ CUPS

2 cups firmly packed fresh basil leaves

¹/₂ cup fresh parsley leaves, preferably flat-leaf

3 medium garlic cloves

¹/₄ cup pine nuts, walnuts, or pistachios

¹/₂ cup extra-virgin olive oil

³/₄ cup shredded dairy-free mozzarella- or Parmesan-style cheese alternative (see Note, page 233)

6 drops basil essential oil

3 drops parsley essential oil (optional)

Freshly ground pink Himalayan salt or sea salt to taste

Freshly ground white pepper to taste

Combine the basil, parsley, garlic, pine nuts, olive oil, cheese-alternative shreds, essential oils, Himalayan salt, and white pepper in a food processor or blender. Cover and process until almost smooth, stopping to scrape down the sides of the bowl as needed.

Serve over cooked vegetables, almond flour pasta, brown rice pasta,* or as a dip. Divide any leftover pesto into containers to freeze or refrigerate.

Portobello Mushrooms Stuffed with Pesto

To watch Mama Z make this delicious stuffed mushroom appetizer, visit EssentialOilsDiet.com.

PREP: 15 MINUTES   COOK: 30 MINUTES   SERVES 8 TO 10

1 (16-ounce) package baby bella mushrooms (about 25 mushrooms)

Olive-oil or coconut-oil cooking spray

Sun-Dried Tomato Pesto (page 239) or another pesto

Shredded dairy-free mozzarella- or Parmesan-style cheese alternative (optional; see Note on page 233)

Preheat the oven to 325°F.

Remove the mushroom stems. Using a spoon or a clean finger, gently remove the gills. Rinse the mushrooms.

Mist a 12 × 12 × 2-inch baking dish with cooking spray and place the mushrooms, top-side up, in the dish. Cook for 15 minutes. Flip the mushrooms over, stuff with the pesto, and top with the cheese-alternative shreds, if desired. Return to the oven for another 15 minutes.

Remove from the oven, let cool slightly, and serve as an appetizer.

Stuffed Portobello Mushroom Salad

Instead of cooling the stuffed mushrooms, serve them over a garden salad as a main dish for 4.

Mama Z's Pumpkin Dip*

PREP: 15 MINUTES   CHILL: 2 HOURS   SERVES 8

2 cups Natural Confectioners' Sugar* (page 262)

1 (15-ounce) can pumpkin puree (see Notes)

1 (8-ounce) container dairy-free almond-milk cream cheese or plain cream cheese–style spread (see Notes)

4 drops cinnamon essential oil

2 drops clove essential oil

1 drop ginger essential oil

Place the confectioners' sugar, pumpkin puree, dairy-free cream cheese, and essential oils in a food processor bowl and process for 1 to 2 minutes, until smooth. Scoop into a serving bowl, cover, and refrigerate for at least 2 hours or up to overnight.

Serve with carrot sticks, apple slices, and/or gluten-free gingersnaps.

NOTES

Don't confuse pureed pumpkin, which is just unsweetened pureed pumpkin, with sweetened pumpkin pie mix. Pureed pumpkin is found in either the baking aisle or the canned goods aisle of the supermarket.

Daiya and Kite Hill offer dairy-free cream cheese.

Mama Z's Hummus

To watch Mama Z make this tasty hummus, visit EssentialOilsDiet.com.

PREP: 15 MINUTES   SERVES 8

3 medium garlic cloves, peeled

2 teaspoons freshly ground pink Himalayan salt or sea salt

1 (15-ounce) can chickpeas, rinsed and drained

3 tablespoons tahini (sesame-seed paste)

3 tablespoons freshly squeezed lemon juice	4 tablespoons extra-virgin olive oil
1 tablespoon raw honey, or 1 dropperful plain liquid stevia	1 drop lemon or lime essential oil
2 tablespoons purified or filtered water	1 teaspoon herbes de Provence, Italian seasoning, or dried rosemary, or 1 tablespoon chopped fresh rosemary

Place the garlic, Himalayan salt, chickpeas, tahini, lemon juice, honey, purified water, 2 tablespoons of the olive oil, and the essential oil (lemon or lime) in the bowl of a food processor or blender. Process until smooth.

Spoon into a serving dish. Top with the herbes de Provence and drizzle with the remaining 2 tablespoons olive oil. Serve as a dip with fresh vegetables and grain-free or almond-flour chips.

Alternatively, place the dip in a 16-ounce airtight container and refrigerate for up to one week, or freeze for a month.

Mama Z's Sun-Dried Tomato Hummus

Add 1/2 cup drained oil-packed sun-dried tomatoes to the other ingredients before processing.

Mama Z's Southwestern Hummus

Use black beans in place of chickpeas and 1 teaspoon chili seasoning instead of the herbes de Provence; add 1 or 2 drops each of cumin and cilantro essential oils along with the lemon essential oil.

Fill in the Gap Nuts

PREP: 15 MINUTES   MAKES 6 CUPS

1 cup sliced or slivered almonds, preferably sprouted

1 cup pecan halves, preferably sprouted

1 cup walnut halves, preferably sprouted

1 cup cashews, preferably sprouted

1 cup pistachios, preferably sprouted

1 cup macadamias, preferably sprouted

1/4 teaspoon freshly ground pink Himalayan salt or sea salt

1/8 to 1/4 teaspoon cayenne pepper

1 to 2 tablespoons raw or manuka honey

Place all the nuts in a large bowl. Add the Himalayan salt and cayenne and stir well. Cover with the honey and toss to mix it throughout. Continue stirring until the honey is well incorporated and barely binds the nuts.

Divide the mixture into twelve 1/2-cup portions and store them separately in 4-ounce canning jars or other small containers.

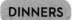

Bok Choy Super Stir-Fry

PREP: 30 MINUTES   COOK: 10 TO 15 MINUTES   SERVES 4

5 ounces fresh baby portobello or shiitake mushrooms, rinsed and stems trimmed

1 small onion, chopped, or 1 tablespoon dried (optional)

2 medium garlic cloves, pressed

1/2 teaspoon ground ginger

1 drop ginger essential oil

2 tablespoons toasted sesame oil

2 tablespoons white wine, dry cooking sherry, or rice wine

2 tablespoons Bragg liquid aminos, or 1 tablespoon gluten-free tamari

1/4 teaspoon freshly ground pink Himalayan salt or sea salt

1/8 teaspoon freshly ground white pepper

1 pound baby bok choy

2 tablespoons raw coconut oil

3 cups freshly chopped stir-fry vegetables, such as carrots, celery, pea pods, bell peppers, broccoli, and/or water chestnuts

Combine the mushrooms and onion, if using, in a shallow dish and add the garlic, ground ginger, ginger essential oil, 1 tablespoon of the sesame oil, white wine, Bragg Aminos, Himalayan salt, and white pepper. Mix well and marinate for 30 minutes.

Meanwhile, separate the bok choy leaves from the stalks. Rinse and thoroughly dry the leaves in a salad spinner. Slice the stalks and leaves horizontally with a serrated knife.

Heat the coconut oil and the 1 remaining tablespoon of sesame oil in a large frying pan or wok over medium to medium-high heat.

Add the stir-fry vegetables and sauté for 5 minutes, tossing several times. Add the bok choy and the marinated mushroom mixture. Cook for another 2 to 5 minutes, until the vegetables are just cooked. Do not let them get soggy.

Serve as is, over a bed of greens or a salad, or with brown basmati rice.

Deluxe Fish Salad

PREP: 25 MINUTES   SERVES 4 TO 6

2 or 3 large eggs (optional)

2 (5- to 7-ounce) cans or dry pouches of wild tuna or wild pink salmon

½ cup grapeseed-oil or avocado-oil vegan mayonnaise

1 tablespoon Dijon or yellow mustard

1 tablespoon apple cider vinegar

1 dropperful plain liquid stevia

2 drops dill essential oil

2 stalks celery, chopped

1 large dill pickle, or 4 small pickles, drained and chopped, or 2 tablespoons pickle relish

2 or 3 Roma tomatoes, quartered, for garnish

2 or 3 sweet bell peppers, sliced, for garnish (optional)

Crumbled pecans or walnuts, for garnish (optional)

Snipped fresh chives, for garnish (optional)

Snipped fresh dill, for garnish (optional)

Paprika to taste

Freshly ground pink Himalayan salt or sea salt to taste

Freshly ground white pepper to taste

If you are using the eggs, place them in a small saucepan and cover with water. Bring the water to a boil, then immediately turn off the heat. Cover and let sit for 15 minutes. Drain the water and run cold water over the eggs for a minute or two. Shell and quarter the eggs. Set aside.

Drain the tuna, gently breaking up the compacted fish, and place it in a large serving dish.

In a small bowl, combine the vegan mayonnaise, mustard, cider vinegar, stevia, and dill essential oil and whisk to blend. Add the celery and dill pickle and toss. Pour the mixture over the fish.

Garnish with the eggs (if using), tomatoes, and, if desired, bell peppers.

If desired, top with the pecans, chives, and dill. Dust with paprika, Himalayan salt, and white pepper. Serve immediately or cover and refrigerate for up to 2 hours before serving.

Deluxe Fish and Pasta Salad*

Cook 2 cups of gluten-free macaroni, fusilli, twists, or shells according to the package directions. Drain, run briefly under cool water, and drain again. Add the pasta to the serving bowl along with the tuna fish, before adding the other ingredients. Use fresh or frozen almond-flour pasta or Miracle Noodle pasta while on Fast Track.

Mama Z's Lasagna

To watch Mama Z make this irresistible Italian
favorite, visit EssentialOilsDiet.com.

PREP: 20 MINUTES   COOK: 70 MINUTES   STAND: 10 TO 15 MINUTES
SERVES 9 TO 12

1 (15-ounce) container unsweetened coconut-milk yogurt substitute

1/2 cup shredded dairy-free Parmesan- or mozzarella-style cheese alternative (see Note, page 233)

2 large eggs, or 1 tablespoon egg replacer plus 2 tablespoons purified or distilled water

2 tablespoons chopped fresh basil, or 2 teaspoons dried

2 tablespoons chopped fresh oregano, or 2 teaspoons dried

2 tablespoons chopped fresh parsley, or 2 teaspoons dried

2 tablespoons chopped fresh thyme, or 2 teaspoons dried

1 drop basil essential oil

1 drop oregano essential oil

1 drop thyme essential oil

1 drop parsley essential oil

8 cups Mama Z's Spaghetti sauce (page 249)

1 (8- to 12-ounce) package brown rice lasagna noodles* (see Note; use frozen almond-flour lasagna or 1 medium eggplant or zucchini, peeled and cut into very thin slices, while on Fast Track)

1 pound fresh or frozen (and defrosted) spinach

2 (7- to 8-ounce) packages shredded dairy-free mozzarella-style cheese alternative (see Note, page 233)

Preheat the oven to 350°F.

In a medium bowl, combine the yogurt substitute, shredded cheese alternative, eggs, 1 tablespoon each of the chopped basil, oregano, parsley, and thyme, and the essential oils.

Place a jelly-roll pan beneath a 9 × 13 × 2-inch baking dish to catch any spills. Spread 1 cup of the spaghetti sauce in the baking dish. Top with one-third of the uncooked lasagna noodles, one-third of the yogurt/cheese mix, one-third of the spinach, and one-third of the remaining spaghetti sauce. Repeat this layer, but this time add half of the mozzarella-style shreds. Repeat with another layer but omit the mozzarella-style shreds. Top with the remaining herbs and the remaining mozzarella-style shreds.

Cut a piece of parchment paper longer than the baking dish (so you can tuck it under on both ends), cover the lasagna, and bake for 1 hour. Remove the parchment paper, return the dish to the oven, and cook for another 10 minutes. Let rest for 10 to 15 minutes before cutting and serving.

NOTE
If you can find fresh almond-flour pasta or brown-rice pasta, go for it. Republic of Pasta sells both fresh and frozen pasta at Whole Foods in the chilled and frozen food aisles. It absorbs less moisture, giving it a nice "tooth." DeBoles is another option. Avoid gluten-free products made from corn or soy.

Slow-Cooker Lasagna

Prepare the sauce and the cheese mixtures as above. Divide the dry noodles into three groups and break each noodle into thirds so that they will fit in the slow cooker. Layer the sauce, yogurt-cheese mixture, spinach, and almond-flour noodles (or vegetable slices) in the slow cooker instead of a baking dish, ending with the mozzarella-style shreds. Cook 4 to 6 hours at Medium or Low, until you can put a fork all the way through the contents to the bottom of the slow cooker.

Meat-Lovers Lasagna*

Mix 1 pound grass-fed ground beef or free-range ground turkey with 1 tablespoon herbes de Provence and cook on the stovetop until browned. Spread one-third of the meat mixture on top of each spinach layer.

Mama Z's Spaghetti

PREP: 20 MINUTES   COOK: 1 TO 2 HOURS   SERVES 6

SAUCE

1 medium onion, chopped, or 1 1/2 tablespoons dried onion

2 medium garlic cloves, pressed

2 tablespoons extra-virgin olive oil, plus more as needed

1 (28-ounce) can or jar Roma tomatoes

1 (28-ounce) can or jar Italian-seasoned tomatoes

1 (6- to 8-ounce) can tomato paste (see Note)

1 cup red wine

2 tablespoons Grade A Dark or C maple syrup* (use 2 dropperfuls liquid stevia while on Fast Track)

2 large carrots, or a handful of baby carrots, and/or 1/2 large beet

1 drop basil essential oil

1 drop oregano essential oil

1 drop thyme essential oil

1 drop parsley essential oil (optional)

1 large bay leaf

1 teaspoon freshly ground pink Himalayan salt or sea salt, plus more as needed

1/2 teaspoon freshly ground white pepper

1 1/2 tablespoons chopped fresh basil, or 1/2 tablespoon dried

1 1/2 tablespoons chopped fresh oregano, or 1/2 tablespoon dried

1 1/2 tablespoons chopped fresh parsley, or 1/2 tablespoon dried

1 1/2 tablespoons chopped fresh thyme, or 1/2 tablespoon dried

PASTA

1 (16-ounce) package fresh, dried, or frozen almond-flour spaghetti (see Note, page 248), or zoodles (spiralized zucchini), seeded if large

1 pound fresh baby spinach, rinsed and spun dry (optional)

In a large pot over low heat, sauté the onion and garlic in the olive oil. When the vegetables are lightly browned, add the Roma and seasoned tomatoes, tomato paste, and red wine, and stir to combine.

Using an immersion blender, blend the sauce to the desired consistency (omit this step if you prefer a chunky sauce). Bring the sauce to a low boil over medium heat and cook, stirring every 15 minutes, until the alcohol from the wine has evaporated, eliminating any acidity, about 60 minutes.

Turn the heat down to low and add the maple syrup, carrots, the essential oils, bay leaf, Himalayan salt, white pepper, and the dried basil, oregano, parsley, and thyme. (If you are using fresh herbs, hold off and add them 10 minutes before the sauce is done.) Let the sauce simmer for at least 1 hour and up to 2 hours for the most robust flavor. Cover and set aside.

Bring a large pot of water to a boil, adding a little Himalayan salt. Add the spaghetti and a little olive oil to prevent the pasta from sticking. Cook the minimum time indicated on the package. Remove from the heat and let the spaghetti sit for a few more minutes, then drain it in a colander. Return the spaghetti to the empty pot with a little more olive oil to prevent it from sticking. (If you're using zoodles, cook them for 2 minutes in boiling water and drain immediately.)

To serve, remove the bay leaf from the sauce and discard. Place a portion of pasta on each plate, followed by a large handful of spinach, if using, and ladle the sauce over it. Alternatively, serve the sauce over a bed of fresh greens or spiralized raw zucchini, or with a fresh side salad.

To store leftovers, mix plenty of sauce with the pasta and top it with extra sauce. To serve, preheat the oven to 325°F and cook, covered, for 15 to 30 minutes. Or refrigerate the sauce for up to a week or freeze it for up to a month to make Mama Z's Lasagna (page 247) another time.

NOTE
If the sauce doesn't thicken up quickly enough, add another can of tomato paste to speed things along.

VARIATION
Instead of one or both cans of tomatoes, use an equivalent amount of pureed garden-fresh, juice-extracted, and cooked-down tomatoes.

Mama Z's Spaghetti with Meat Sauce*

Brown 1 pound grass-fed ground beef or free-range ground turkey with the onion and garlic, then continue with the recipe.

Garden-Fresh Quinoa Salad

PREP: 20 MINUTES   CHILL: 2 HOURS   SERVES 6 TO 8

1 cup quinoa, cooked and cooled

1 (14-ounce) can chickpeas, rinsed and drained

1 large ripe tomato, sliced

1 cup peeled, seeded, and diced cucumbers

1/2 cup sliced green onions, or 2 tablespoons dried onion

2 medium garlic cloves, pressed

1/4 cup chopped fresh parsley leaves

2 tablespoons chopped fresh basil or mint leaves

1/4 cup extra-virgin olive oil

1/4 cup freshly squeezed lemon juice

1/4 teaspoon freshly ground white pepper

1 teaspoon freshly ground pink Himalayan salt or sea salt

2 drops lemon essential oil

2 drops parsley essential oil

Fresh mint leaves, for garnish

Combine the quinoa, chickpeas, tomatoes, cucumbers, green onions, garlic, parsley, basil, olive oil, lemon juice, white pepper, Himalayan salt, and essential oils in a large bowl, and gently mix. Garnish with mint leaves. Chill 2 hours and serve.

South of the Border Casserole

PREP: 20 MINUTES   COOK: 30 TO 60 MINUTES   SERVES 8

½ cup raw brown basmati rice

Butter or raw coconut oil

1 (16-ounce) can vegetarian refried black beans

3 large Hass avocados, peeled and pitted

3 tablespoons freshly squeezed lime or lemon juice

3 drops lime essential oil

3 drops cilantro essential oil

8 ounces grapeseed-oil or avocado-oil vegan mayonnaise

2 tablespoons Mama Z's Taco Seasoning (page 257), or preservative-free taco seasoning such as Primal Palate organic

1 (4-ounce) can fire-roasted green chile peppers, drained and chopped

3 medium or 5 small Roma tomatoes, chopped

¾ cup pitted and sliced black olives, plus more (optional) for serving

2 cups shredded dairy-free Cheddar-style cheese alternative (see Note, page 228)

Preheat the oven to 350°F.

In a small saucepan set over high heat, bring 1 cup water to a boil, reduce the heat to a low simmer, and add the rice and a tablespoon of butter. Cover and cook for 10 to 14 minutes. (It can be slightly undercooked as it will absorb more liquid while it bakes.)

Spread an even layer of the refried beans on the bottom of an 8 × 8 × 2-inch baking dish. Cover with the cooked rice. Place the avocados in a food processor or a bowl. Add the lime juice and the essential oils and blend or mash until well combined. Spread the mixture evenly on top of the rice.

Blend the vegan mayonnaise and the taco seasoning together in a bowl or food processor. Spread evenly over the avocado layer. In the food processor, blend the chiles and tomatoes together and layer them evenly over the taco seasoning, followed with a layer of black olives. Top it off with the Cheddar-style shreds.

Bake for 30 minutes to 1 hour, depending on how crisp you want the cheese. Serve with gluten-free taco chips, extra olives, and sliced avocado, or over a salad.

APPETIZER VARIATION
Serve with carrot and celery sticks, or organic corn chips*. (Serves 16)

Colorful Kale Salad

PREP: 15 MINUTES   CHILL: 1 HOUR   COOK: 30 MINUTES   SERVES 4

1 cup cooked quinoa or brown rice

1/2 cup raisins

1/2 cup green or red grapes, halved lengthwise

6 cups (8 ounces) shredded kale, measured after stems and spines are removed

1 (15.5-ounce) can chickpeas, black beans, or lentils, rinsed and drained

1 cup shredded carrots, beets, or zucchini, or a combination

1/2 cup shredded red or green cabbage

1/2 cup chopped walnuts or pecans (optional)

1 cup Vegan Greek Dressing (page 256)

In a large bowl (preferably one with a lid or cover), mix together the quinoa, raisins, grapes, shredded kale, chickpeas, carrots, cabbage, and walnuts, if using.

Pour the cup of dressing over the salad. If the bowl has a lid, cover the bowl, shake the salad thoroughly, then transfer it to a serving bowl. Alternatively, toss the salad and serve.

SAUCES, DRESSINGS, CONDIMENTS, AND BUTTERS

Basil Butter

PREP: 5 MINUTES   CHILL: 1 HOUR   MAKES 1/2 CUP

4 ounces (1 stick) butter, at room temperature

1 tablespoon finely chopped fresh basil, or 1 teaspoon dried

3 drops basil essential oil

In a small bowl, mix the softened butter with the basil and essential oil. Cover and refrigerate for an hour, until ready to serve.

Dill Butter

Substitute the same amount of fresh or dried dill for the basil and use dill essential oil.

When making flavored butters, I recommend that you match the essential oil and herb, so basil with basil essential oil, dill with dill essential oil, and so on.

Family Favorite Italian Dressing

PREP: 5 MINUTES   STAND: 15 TO 30 MINUTES   MAKES ROUGHLY 10 TABLESPOONS

1/4 cup apple cider vinegar

6 tablespoons extra-virgin olive oil

1 medium garlic clove, pressed

1/2 teaspoon chopped fresh marjoram

1 teaspoon chopped fresh basil

1 teaspoon chopped fresh oregano

1 drop marjoram essential oil

1 drop basil essential oil

1 drop oregano essential oil

1/2 teaspoon freshly ground pink Himalayan salt or sea salt

1/4 teaspoon freshly ground white pepper

Combine the cider vinegar, olive oil, garlic, fresh herbs, essential oils, Himalayan salt, and white pepper in a pint jar; tighten the top and shake vigorously. Alternatively, whisk the ingredients in a medium bowl or use an immersion blender to thoroughly mix the ingredients.

Let the jar sit for 15 to 30 minutes so the flavors develop before dressing a salad.

VARIATION

Top fresh greens with grilled skewered veggies, tempeh, or beef, and drizzle the dressing over them for a one-dish dinner. Or use the dressing as a marinade.

Safety note: Discard any dressing used to marinate beef or other animal products.

Dreamy, Creamy Italian Dressing

PREP: 5 MINUTES   MAKES 20 TABLESPOONS

1 cup grapeseed-oil or avocado-oil vegan mayonnaise

1/2 small yellow or red onion, finely chopped

2 tablespoons red wine vinegar or balsamic vinegar

1 tablespoon coconut sugar* or 1/2 tablespoon raw honey* (use 1 dropperful plain liquid stevia while on Fast Track)

3/4 teaspoon herbes de Provence or dried Italian seasoning

1/4 teaspoon freshly ground pink Himalayan salt or sea salt

1/4 teaspoon garlic powder

1/8 teaspoon freshly ground white pepper

1 drop basil essential oil

1 drop lavender essential oil

1 drop rosemary essential oil

1 drop tarragon essential oil (optional)

1 drop thyme essential oil

Place the vegan mayonnaise, onion, vinegar, coconut sugar, herbes de Provence, Himalayan salt, garlic powder, white pepper, and the essential oils in a pint jar. Tighten the lid, making sure it is secure, and shake vigorously. Alternatively, blend the ingredients in a small bowl using a wire whisk or a small handheld immersion blender.

Vegan Greek Dressing

PREP: 10 MINUTES   MAKES 2 CUPS

1 cup apple cider vinegar

1/2 cup extra-virgin olive oil

1/2 cup Spanish olive oil

1 tablespoon coconut sugar* or
2 tablespoons raw honey* or
Grade A Dark or C maple syrup*
(use 2 dropperfuls liquid stevia while
on Fast Track)

1 tablespoon freshly ground pink
Himalayan salt or sea salt

4 to 6 medium garlic cloves, pressed

1 tablespoon freshly squeezed lemon
or lime juice

2 teaspoons herbes de Provence or
Greek seasoning, or 1/2 teaspoon
each dried basil, oregano, parsley, and
thyme

1 teaspoon yellow or Dijon mustard

1/2 teaspoon crushed red pepper flakes

1/2 teaspoon freshly ground white
pepper

2 drops lemon essential oil

2 drops lime essential oil

In a glass jar with a tight-fitting lid, combine the cider vinegar, both olive oils, coconut sugar, Himalayan salt, garlic, lemon juice, herbes de Provence, mustard, red pepper flakes, white pepper, and the essential oils. Tighten the lid, making sure it is secure, and shake vigorously. Use the dressing immediately and refrigerate any leftovers. It can also be used as a marinade, but do not then use it as a dressing on the completed dish.

Paradise Fruit Spicy Salsa

PREP: 10 TO 15 MINUTES   MAKES 6 TO 8 CUPS

5 freestone peaches, peeled and
pitted (see Notes)

1 small cantaloupe (about 1 pound),
peeled and seeded

12 ounces mango, peeled and pit
removed

12 ounces strawberries, stemmed

1 cup pineapple cubes

Freshly squeezed juice of 2 limes

1/4 cup fresh cilantro leaves

2 teaspoons coconut crystals* (use
2 dropperfuls liquid stevia while on the
Fast Track)

1/2 teaspoon freshly ground pink
Himalayan salt or sea salt

3 fresh jalapeño peppers (see Notes)

3 fresh banana peppers (see Notes)

1 fresh cayenne pepper (see Notes)

1 fresh habanero pepper (see Notes)

2 drops cilantro essential oil

2 drops lime essential oil

2 drops lemon essential oil

Combine the peaches, cantaloupe, mango, strawberries, pineapple cubes, lime juice, cilantro, coconut crystals, Himalayan salt, jalapeños, banana peppers, cayenne pepper, habanero, and the essential oils in a food processor. Pulse until the ingredients reach the desired consistency, anywhere from chunky to smooth.

Depending upon the size of your processor, you may need to make this in batches. If so, combine the batches together in a large bowl.

Use immediately, or portion into small glass or freezer-safe containers and refrigerate or freeze.

NOTES

To peel a peach, dip it in boiling water for 20 seconds, then allow it to cool slightly; the skin should come off easily.

To prepare the peppers without getting the volatile oils on your hands, snip off the tip with a pair of scissors and cut through the pepper several times. Remove all or most of the seeds and pulp; if you prefer a less spicy salsa, remove all the seeds and pulp, using kitchen gloves.

Mama Z's Taco Seasoning

PREP: 5 MINUTES   MAKES ¹/2 CUP

2 tablespoons chili powder

2 tablespoons ground cumin

1 tablespoon plus 1 teaspoon freshly ground white pepper

2 teaspoons paprika

1 teaspoon garlic powder

1 teaspoon dried oregano

1 teaspoon freshly ground pink Himalayan salt or sea salt

In a small bowl, mix the chili powder, cumin, white pepper, paprika, garlic powder, oregano, and Himalayan salt. Store the mixture in a glass jar with a tight-fitting lid placed away from the light. Use the seasoning to add a south-of-the-border flavor to eggs and many other dishes.

Mama Z's Taco Dip

Mix 2 tablespoons of the taco seasoning with a cup of grapeseed-oil or avocado-oil vegan mayonnaise.

Lemon Abundance Tea Bread*

To watch Mama Z make this delectable
treat, visit EssentialOilsDiet.com.

PREP: 25 MINUTES   COOK: 1 HOUR   STAND: 10 MINUTES   SERVES 6

Olive-oil or coconut-oil cooking spray

1¼ cups gluten-free all-purpose flour, plus more for the pan

½ cup (1 stick) butter, at room temperature, or raw coconut oil

1 teaspoon plain liquid stevia, or 1 cup coconut sugar

2 large eggs

¼ cup coconut flour

1 teaspoon aluminum-free baking powder

½ teaspoon freshly ground pink Himalayan salt or sea salt

½ cup canned full-fat unsweetened coconut milk

1 tablespoon grated lemon zest

1 tablespoon freshly squeezed lemon juice

3 to 6 drops lemon essential oil

DRIZZLE TOPPING

1 rounded cup Natural Confectioners' Sugar (page 262)

1 tablespoon freshly squeezed lemon juice

3 drops lemon essential oil

1 tablespoon grated lemon zest

1½ teaspoons to 1 tablespoon raw honey

Preheat the oven to 350°F. Mist an 8 × 4-inch loaf pan, 2 smaller loaf pans, or 12-muffin cup pans with cooking spray and dust with flour. If using muffin papers, do not mist or flour.

In a large bowl, beat the butter with an electric mixer at medium speed until creamy. Gradually add the stevia, beating until light and fluffy. Add the eggs, one at a time, mixing thoroughly.

In a medium bowl, stir together the flour, coconut flour, baking powder, and Himalayan salt. Add the flour mixture to the creamed mixture alternately with the coconut milk, beating at low speed just until blended, beginning and ending with the flour mixture. Stir in the lemon zest, the lemon juice, and 3 to 6 drops of the lemon essential oil, depending upon how intense you want the lemon flavor.

Spoon the batter into the prepared pan. Bake the larger loaf pan for about 1 hour, or until a wooden toothpick inserted in the center of the loaf comes out clean. (Halve the time for the smaller loaf pans, but check them at 20 minutes; mini muffins take 15 to 20 minutes.) Let the tea bread cool in the pan for 10 minutes. Remove the bread from the pan and let it cool completely on a wire rack.

For the drizzle topping: Place the confectioners' sugar in a medium bowl and add 1^1/$_2$ teaspoons of the lemon juice and the essential oil, stirring until smooth. Add up to another 1^1/$_2$ teaspoons lemon juice, as needed, but don't make the mixture too runny. Place the cooled bread on a serving plate. Spoon the mixture evenly over the top, letting any excess drip down the sides. Stir together the lemon zest and honey to taste; sprinkle on top of the loaf, and serve.

Lemon-Almond Tea Bread*

Stir ^{1}/$_2$ teaspoon pure almond extract into the batter and bake as above.

Brown Rice Pudding*

PREP: 20 MINUTES   COOK: 1 HOUR   SERVES 6 TO 8

1 cup uncooked brown rice or brown basmati rice

Butter or raw coconut oil

1 (13.5-ounce) can full-fat unsweetened coconut milk (1½ cups)

½ cup raisins or currants

¼ cup raw coconut oil

1 tablespoon egg replacer, or 2 large eggs

1 tablespoon pure vanilla extract

1 teaspoon freshly ground Himalayan salt or sea salt

1 teaspoon ground Ceylon cinnamon, plus extra for topping

½ teaspoon pumpkin pie spice mix (see Note), plus extra for topping

3 to 4 dropperfuls vanilla-flavored liquid stevia, or 1 tablespoon Grade A Dark or C maple syrup, or 1½ teaspoons coconut sugar

⅓ cup chopped walnuts or pecans (optional)

In a medium saucepan set over high heat, bring 2 cups water to a boil, reduce the heat to a low simmer, and add the brown rice and some butter. Cover and cook the rice for 20 to 30 minutes, until the water has been absorbed and the rice is fluffy; brown basmati rice will take only 10 to 14 minutes. (It can be slightly undercooked as it will absorb more liquid when it is baking in the oven.)

Meanwhile, preheat the oven to 350°F.

Add the coconut milk, raisins, coconut oil, egg replacer, vanilla, Himalayan salt, cinnamon, pumpkin pie spice, stevia, and walnuts (if using) to the cooked rice in the saucepan. Mix well.

Transfer the rice mixture to a 1½-quart baking dish. Top with a sprinkle of cinnamon and pumpkin pie spice. Bake for about 1 hour, or until the pudding is firm.

Let the pudding cool for 30 minutes, or serve warm with Mama Z's Vanilla Ice Cream (page 263) or Coconut Whipped Cream (page 262).

NOTE
Pumpkin pie spice is a blend of cinnamon, ginger, allspice, and nutmeg. You'll find it at Whole Foods and most other well-stocked supermarkets.

Crustless Cranberry Pie

PREP: 20 MINUTES   COOK: 40 MINUTES   SERVES 8

Coconut-oil or olive-oil cooking spray

2 large eggs, or 1 tablespoon egg replacer plus 2 tablespoons purified or distilled water

1 cup gluten-free all-purpose flour* (use almond flour during Fast Track)

1/4 teaspoon freshly ground pink Himalayan salt or sea salt

2 cups fresh or frozen cranberries

1/2 cup chopped walnuts

1/2 cup (1 stick) butter, melted

1 teaspoon pure almond extract

4 dropperfuls liquid stevia

1 or 2 drops orange essential oil

Preheat the oven to 350°F. Mist a 9-inch pie pan with cooking spray.

In a medium bowl, beat the eggs. Alternatively, mix the egg replacer with the water in a medium bowl.

In a separate bowl, combine the flour and Himalayan salt. Stir in the cranberries and walnuts and toss to coat. Stir in the melted butter, beaten eggs, almond extract, liquid stevia, and orange essential oil. (If you are using frozen cranberries, the mixture will be very thick.) Spread the batter evenly in the prepared pan.

Bake for about 40 minutes, or until a toothpick inserted near the center comes out clean. Serve warm with Coconut Whipped Cream (page 262) or Mama Z's Vanilla Ice Cream (page 263).

Natural Confectioners' Sugar*

PREP: 5 MINUTES   MAKES 4 CUPS

4 rounded cups honey granules, maple sugar, or coconut sugar

6 to 8 teaspoons arrowroot or non-GMO cornstarch

Place the honey granules and arrowroot in a food processor or blender and process until well blended. Store in a glass jar at room temperature. Use as directed in desserts and dips.

Coconut Whipped Cream

PREP: 5 MINUTES   CHILL: 3 TO 4 HOURS   SERVES 8 TO 10

1 (13.5-ounce) can full-fat unsweetened coconut milk (1^1/$_2$ cups), refrigerated overnight

1 tablespoon pure vanilla extract

2 to 3 dropperfuls vanilla-flavored liquid stevia, or 1 teaspoon maple syrup or raw honey*

After the can of coconut milk has chilled in the refrigerator overnight, turn the can upside down the next morning, open it, and drain off the liquid (save it to use later in a smoothie).

Place the coconut cream left in the can in the bowl of a stand mixer fitted with the paddle or whisk attachment, and add the vanilla and stevia to taste. Beat until fluffy.

Chill in the refrigerator, covered, for 3 to 4 hours before serving.

Mama Z's Vanilla Ice Cream

PREP: 10 MINUTES   CHILL: 30 MINUTES   MAKES 3 CUPS

1 (13.5-ounce) can full-fat unsweetened coconut milk (1¹/₂ cups)

1¹/₂ cups unsweetened vanilla-flavored almond or coconut milk beverage

1 tablespoon pure vanilla extract

5 to 6 dropperfuls vanilla-flavored liquid stevia, or ³/₄ cup coconut crystals* or raw honey*

Pinch of freshly ground pink Himalayan salt or sea salt

1 tablespoon egg replacer plus ¹/₄ cup purified or distilled water

¹/₄ teaspoon ground vanilla bean, or scraped seeds of ¹/₂ vanilla bean

Place the interior bowl of an automatic ice cream maker in the freezer for at least 12 hours.

Place the canned coconut milk in a blender. Add enough almond milk beverage to reach the 3-cup mark. Add the vanilla, stevia, Himalayan salt, egg replacer and purified water, and vanilla bean. Blend well.

Place the interior bowl and the paddle in the electric ice cream maker. Turn the machine on and pour in the contents of the blender. Let the ice cream maker run for about 30 minutes, or until the ice cream reaches your preferred consistency.

Serve immediately or keep it in the interior bowl in the freezer.

Mama Z's Peppermint Stick Ice Cream

Add either 1 tablespoon of pure peppermint extract or 2 to 5 drops of peppermint essential oil to the blender.

Mama Z's Chocolate-Almond Ice Cream

Replace the tablespoon of vanilla extract with 2 teaspoons pure vanilla extract and 1 teaspoon pure almond extract; add ¹/₄ cup cacao powder to the mixture before blending. Stir in ¹/₂ cup sliced or slivered almonds before freezing the mixture.

Superfood Peppermint Patties

PREP: 30 MINUTES   CHILL: 2 HOURS   MAKES 20 TO 24 PATTIES

2¹/2 cups raw coconut oil, at room temperature

¹/2 cup raw honey* (use 6 dropperfuls liquid stevia while on Fast Track)

2 or 3 drops peppermint essential oil, or 1 teaspoon pure peppermint extract

3 (3-ounce) dark chocolate bars, minimum 72% cacao

In a medium bowl and using a wooden spoon, mix together 2 cups of the coconut oil, the honey, and the peppermint essential oil until well blended. Form the mixture into 20 to 24 patties and place them on a large parchment paper–covered plate. Alternatively, put each patty in a compartment of a mini-muffin pan. Place the patties in the freezer to harden, 20 to 30 minutes. Once they are firm, remove them to a ziplock plastic bag.

Meanwhile, in a saucepan set over medium heat, melt the chocolate bars and the remaining ¹/2 cup coconut oil. Remove the pan from the heat and allow to cool for 5 to 10 minutes. Dip each frozen patty into the chocolate mixture to cover and return it to the parchment-covered plate or mini-muffin pan. Return the plate or pan to the freezer until the chocolate has hardened, at least 1¹/2 hours. Store the patties in a freezer bag in the freezer indefinitely.

Dark Chocolate–Peppermint Brownies*

PREP: 15 MINUTES   COOK: 18 TO 25 MINUTES   STAND: 10 MINUTES

MAKES 32 BROWNIES

1/4 cup raw coconut oil, softened, plus more for greasing the pan

2/3 cup coconut sugar*

1/2 cup Grade A Dark or C maple syrup* or raw honey* (use 6 dropperfuls liquid stevia while on Fast Track)

1/2 cup (1 stick) butter, melted

2 tablespoons purified or distilled water

2 large eggs, beaten

1 tablespoon pure vanilla extract

1 cup gluten-free all-purpose flour

1/3 cup coconut flour

3/4 cup unsweetened cacao or dark cocoa powder

1/2 teaspoon aluminum-free baking powder

1/4 teaspoon freshly ground pink Himalayan salt or sea salt

2 to 5 drops peppermint essential oil, or 1 teaspoon pure peppermint extract

Preheat the oven to 350°F. Grease a 13 × 9 × 2-inch baking pan.

Combine the coconut sugar, maple syrup, butter, coconut oil, and purified water in a large bowl. Stir in the eggs and vanilla.

In another bowl, combine the flour, coconut flour, cacao, baking powder, and Himalayan salt. Add the dry ingredients to the wet ones and mix well. Stir in the peppermint essential oil, using fewer drops if you prefer a mild peppermint flavor or more if you want full intensity. Spread the mixture evenly in the prepared pan and bake for 18 to 25 minutes, until a toothpick comes out clean. Remove from the oven and allow to cool in the pan for 10 minutes.

Cut into 32 pieces. Serve with Coconut Whipped Cream (page 262) or Mama Z's Vanilla Ice Cream (page 263). Place in airtight container and store in fridge or freezer (for longer).

MAMA Z TIP

Don't overbeat the batter or the brownies will not fluff up.

Dr. Z's Black Bean–Chocolate Brownies

PREP: 30 MINUTES   COOK: 30 TO 45 MINUTES   STAND: 15 MINUTES

MAKES 16 BROWNIES

Coconut-oil or olive-oil cooking spray, for greasing the pan

3 large eggs

1/2 cup canned full-fat unsweetened coconut milk, plus more as needed

1/4 cup raw coconut oil, melted

1 teaspoon pure vanilla extract

3 dropperfuls vanilla-flavored liquid stevia

1 (13-ounce) can black beans, rinsed and drained

1/2 cup gluten-free all-purpose flour* (use almond flour while on Fast Track)

1/2 cup raw cacao powder

1/2 cup coconut sugar* (use 2 dropperfuls liquid stevia while on Fast Track)

Pinch of freshly ground Himalayan pink salt or sea salt

Preheat the oven to 350°F. Mist an 8 × 8 × 2-inch baking pan with cooking spray.

In a large bowl, beat the eggs. Add the coconut milk, coconut oil, vanilla, and stevia, and blend well. Gently fold in the black beans.

In a medium bowl, mix the flour, cacao powder, coconut sugar (omit if you are on the Fast Track), and Himalayan salt. Fold the dry ingredients into the wet ingredients; you may need to add up to 1/4 cup more coconut milk to get perfect brownie consistency. (Gluten-free flours tend to be heavier and require more liquids than wheat flour.)

Pour the batter into the prepared pan and bake for 30 minutes before testing for doneness by inserting a toothpick in the center; continue to bake and test again at 5-minute intervals until the toothpick comes out clean, which could be up to 45 minutes, depending on the flour used. Don't overbake the brownies.

Let the brownies cool in the pan for 15 minutes, then cut them into 16 pieces and place in an airtight container. Store in the refrigerator.

Black Bean-Carob Brownies

Replace the cacao with carob powder.

Other Variations

Stir some unsweetened coconut flakes or chopped walnuts into the batter before baking. You will likely also have to add a *little* extra coconut oil and milk, but a little goes a long way.

Dr. Z's Chocolate-Avocado Puddin'

PREP: 30 MINUTES   SERVES 8

3 Hass avocados, peeled and pitted

1/4 to 1 cup canned full-fat, unsweetened coconut milk

1 teaspoon pure vanilla extract

1/2 cup raw cacao powder

2 dropperfuls vanilla-flavored liquid stevia

Place the avocados in the bowl of a food processor. Add 1/4 cup of the coconut milk, vanilla, cacao powder, and stevia. Blend until smooth, making sure to scrape down the sides of the processor several times with a silicone spatula. Add additional coconut milk as needed to create the desired consistency.

Serve immediately; keep any leftovers, covered, in the fridge for up to three days.

Mama Z's Triple Lemon Bars*

PREP: 10 TO 15 MINUTES   COOK: 50 MINUTES   MAKES 32 BARS

CRUST

1½ cups gluten-free all-purpose flour

½ cup coconut flour

½ cup coconut sugar

¼ teaspoon freshly ground pink Himalayan salt or sea salt

½ cup (1 stick) cold unsalted butter, cut into pieces, or ½ cup raw coconut oil

½ cup raw coconut oil

FILLING

4 large eggs

6 tablespoons gluten-free all-purpose flour

½ cup coconut sugar

1 teaspoon aluminum-free baking powder

Pinch of freshly ground pink Himalayan salt or sea salt

1 cup Grade A Dark or C maple syrup or raw honey

½ cup purified or distilled water or unsweetened coconut milk beverage

½ cup freshly squeezed lemon juice

3 drops lemon essential oil

1 tablespoon Natural Confectioners' Sugar (optional; page 262)

Finely grated lemon zest, for garnish (optional)

Preheat the oven to 350° F.

Make the crust: In a large bowl, mix together both flours, the coconut sugar, and Himalayan salt. Using a knife, cut the butter and coconut oil into the dry ingredients to form a dough with a fine-crumb consistency. Press the mixture in an even layer in the bottom of a 9 × 13 × 2-inch pan. Bake for 20 minutes, until pale golden.

Meanwhile, make the filling: In a medium bowl, beat the eggs.

In a separate medium bowl, stir together the flour, coconut sugar, baking powder, and Himalayan salt.

Add the flour mixture to the eggs and stir until smooth. Gradually stir in the maple syrup, distilled water, lemon juice, and lemon essential oil. Pour the mixture over the baked crust and return to the oven.

Bake for about 30 minutes, or until set. Cool completely (15 to 30 minutes) before sifting the Natural Confectioners' Sugar over the top, if desired. Garnish with lemon zest, if desired. Cut into 32 pieces. Place in airtight container and store in fridge or freezer (for longer).

Using two or three different sweeteners, as you can once you are no longer in the Fast Track, gives body as well as a more full-bodied flavor. If you don't have access to all these sweeteners, use more of one or two of the others.

Mama Z's Triple Orange Bars*

Substitute freshly squeezed orange juice for the lemon juice, orange essential oil for the lemon oil, and orange zest for the lemon zest.

Keep freshly squeezed lemon or lime juice in the fridge to speed up recipe prep.

Our Carrot Wedding Cake*

PREP: 5 TO 10 MINUTES   COOK: 45 MINUTES
MAKES 1 SHEET CAKE THAT SERVES 18

Coconut-oil or olive-oil cooking spray, for greasing the pan

1/2 cup (1 stick) butter, softened, or raw coconut oil

1/2 cup raw organic coconut oil

1 1/2 cups raw honey

4 large eggs

2 1/4 cups gluten-free all-purpose flour

3/4 cup coconut flour

2 teaspoons baking soda

2 teaspoons ground Ceylon cinnamon

3 cups grated carrots

1 cup chopped pecans, walnuts, or a combo (optional)

3 drops Immunity Blend (see Immune-Boosting Matcha Latte, page 216)

Easy "Cream Cheese" Frosting* (page 271)

Preheat the oven to 300°F. Mist a 9 × 13 × 2-inch pan with cooking spray.

In a large mixing bowl, thoroughly blend the butter, coconut oil, honey, and eggs.

In another bowl, combine both flours, the baking soda, and cinnamon. Sift 1 1/2 cups of the flour mixture over the egg mixture. Stir, then add the remaining sifted flour mixture and stir until well blended. Fold in the carrots, nuts (if using), and Immunity Blend.

Spread the batter in the prepared pan and bake for about 45 minutes, or until a toothpick inserted near the center comes out clean. Remove the cake from the oven and let it cool on a wire rack before frosting.

Easy "Cream Cheese" Frosting*

PREP: 5 MINUTES   MAKES ENOUGH FOR A 9 × 13 × 2-INCH SHEET CAKE

1 (8-ounce) container dairy-free cream-cheese substitute (see Notes, page 242), at room temperature

1/3 cup raw honey

1 tablespoon pure vanilla extract

Ground Ceylon cinnamon

Pumpkin pie spice (see Notes, page 242)

In a blender or food processor, combine the dairy-free cream cheese, honey, and vanilla. Blend until smooth and fluffy. Top with cinnamon and/or pumpkin pie spice. Store in the refrigerator for up to a week.

Easy Lemon Pie with Essential Oils*

PREP: 20 MINUTES   CHILL: 6 HOURS   SERVES 8

Lemon Dip with Essential Oils* (page 238)

Cookie Crumb Piecrust* (page 272)

Chill the prepared lemon dip in the refrigerator for at least 6 hours or overnight. Pour the entire cold dip into the cooled piecrust. Serve immediately or store in the refrigerator for up to a week.

Cookie Crumb Piecrust*

PREP: 10 MINUTES   COOK: 10 MINUTES   STAND: 20 MINUTES

MAKES ONE 9-INCH CRUST

Coconut-oil or olive-oil cooking spray

1½ cups crumbs from gluten-free coconut sugar cookies, such as Simple Mills Crunchy Cinnamon or Crunchy Toasted Pecan Cookies

¼ cup (½ stick) butter or raw coconut oil, melted

¼ teaspoon freshly ground pink Himalayan salt or sea salt

Preheat the oven to 350°F. Mist a 9-inch glass pie pan with cooking spray.

In a food processor, combine the cookie crumbs, butter, and salt and process until evenly mixed. Put aside 2 to 3 tablespoons of the crumb mixture for the topping. Press the remaining mixture firmly and evenly against the bottom and sides of the pie pan.

Bake for 10 minutes. Allow to cool on a wire rack, about 20 minutes, before adding the pie filling.

Easy Pumpkin Pie with Essential Oils*

PREP: 10 MINUTES   CHILL: 6 HOURS   SERVES 8

Mama Z's Pumpkin Dip* (page 242)

Cookie Crumb Piecrust* (above)

Chill the prepared pumpkin dip in the refrigerator for at least 6 hours or overnight. Pour the entire cold dip into the cooled piecrust. Serve immediately or store in the refrigerator for up to a week.

ESSENTIAL OILS REMEDIES

The essential oil remedies that follow have been formulated to help you shed excess pounds, burn fat, and approach weight loss on a fundamental level—by treating the primary root causes: elevated blood sugar, gut and digestive disorders, chronic inflammation, stress, and sleep issues.

These recipes require a carrier oil that properly dilutes the essential oils to prevent any skin sensitization and to help avoid adverse reactions. For our non–roller bottle recipes, our favorite carrier is a mixture we call Mama Z's Oil Base (page 274). Prepare a batch and keep it on hand to speed up the process of making the most of your DIY remedies. Note that because Mama Z's Oil Base contains regular coconut oil, it will harden at room temperature, so you'll want to avoid this as a carrier for your roller bottle recipes. Fractionated coconut oil (see page 117), sweet almond oil, and jojoba oil all work great in roller bottles.

Mama Z's Oil Base

This versatile base can be used to formulate multiple healing salves and balms. This recipe makes a lot. Divide all ingredients in half or quarters to make a smaller batch.

54 ounces raw coconut oil

16 ounces sweet almond oil

8 ounces jojoba oil

4 ounces vitamin E oil

Essential oil of your choice (see Notes)

SUPPLIES

Quart- or pint-size widemouthed mason jars or other glass containers with lids

1. To preserve the nutritional content of the coconut oil, liquefy it by immersing the jar in a bowl or saucepan of warm (not boiling) water for a few minutes. Do not heat it directly on the stovetop.

2. In a large bowl or cooking pot, combine the melted coconut oil with the sweet almond, jojoba, and vitamin E oils. Add your choice of essential oil. If desired, use a wire whisk to reach a smoother "whipped" consistency. Alternatively, you can blend them in a blender.

3. Pour the mixture into mason jars and tightly close the lids. Store in a cool (see Notes), dark place for up to two years. The saturated fats in the coconut oil won't spoil, but the sweet almond oil may get stale if not properly stored.

NOTES

To make your own blends, use 6 to 8 drops of essential oils for every ounce of the base.

Coconut oil has a melting point of 76°F. Depending on the temperature in your house, the base may revert to a solid or semisolid state. To reliquefy it, rub some in your hands or place the container close to a heating vent or in warm water.

ESSENTIAL OILS FOR WEIGHT LOSS

In addition to treating the root causes of weight gain, essential oils can directly trigger your body to burn fat, curb hunger, and treat food addiction. These recipes are a great place to start. Remember, you can customize them to your liking and according to the supplies that you have on hand.

Fat-Burning Roll-On

From The Healing Power of Essential Oils

4 drops lime essential oil

3 drops peppermint essential oil

3 drops grapefruit essential oil

2 drops cypress essential oil

1 drop eucalyptus essential oil

1 drop cinnamon bark essential oil

Carrier oil of your choice (Mama Z's Oil Base, page 274, or fractionated coconut, jojoba, or sweet almond oil) to fill a roller bottle

SUPPLIES
10-ml glass roller bottle

1. Drop the essential oils into the roller bottle.

2. Fill the bottle with your favorite carrier oil.

3. Shake vigorously for 10 seconds.

4. Three or four times a week, apply the oil over problem areas (see Note), such as the stomach, back of the thighs, and undersides of the upper arms, after you shower.

NOTE
Test this first on the back of your hand or bottoms of your feet to make sure your body responds well to the blend. Discontinue use immediately if irritation occurs.

Fat-Burning Wrap

From The Healing Power of Essential Oils

Fat-Burning Roll-On (page 275)

SUPPLIES
1 yard muslin fabric, cut into strips large enough to cover the body part you want to treat, but small enough to be manageable

Plastic wrap

1. Right before bed, liberally apply the Fat-Burning Roll-On over any areas of concern.

2. Wrap each area of the body individually with muslin.

3. Cover the fabric with two or three layers of plastic wrap.

4. When you wake up, unwrap each area and wipe yourself down with a towel before showering.

Cut-Your-Cravings Diffuser Blend

1 drop cinnamon essential oil

2 drops black pepper essential oil

2 drops peppermint essential oil

SUPPLIES
Diffuser

1. Fill the diffuser with water as directed in the manufacturer's instructions.

2. Add the essential oils to the water (see Note).

3. When cravings for unhealthy foods occur, turn on the diffuser, sit down, and relax for a few minutes. Be sure to take intentional slow, deep breaths.

4. Turn off the diffuser when your cravings cease.

NOTE
You can keep this mixture in the diffuser and use it daily until it is empty.

Quit Sticks

This recipe was formulated for smokers but works equally well for people with food addictions.

20 drops black pepper essential oil

10 drops grapefruit essential oil

5 drops peppermint essential oil

5 drops orange essential oil

5 drops cinnamon bark essential oil

Edible carrier oil (see Note)

SUPPLIES

1 (1-ounce) glass measuring cup or shot glass

50 to 75 toothpicks (enough to fill your glass)

Clean plate or baking sheet

Glass toothpick container

1. Drop the essential oils into the measuring cup.

2. Fill the cup three-quarters full with the carrier oil and stir.

3. Place the toothpicks in the cup and let them soak overnight.

4. Remove the toothpicks and let them dry on the clean plate or baking sheet.

5. When cravings for unhealthy foods arise, suck on a toothpick.

6. Store the "sticks" in a glass toothpick container.

NOTE
Use an edible carrier oil that won't harden, such as extra-virgin olive oil, grape-seed oil, or avocado oil.

BALANCE BLOOD SUGAR AND BEAT TYPE 2 DIABETES

In chapter 6, we discussed the power of essential oils to help balance blood sugar, reduce lipid accumulation, and enhance insulin sensitivity. Fourteen different oils, each of which appears in one of the following recipes, can help you achieve these goals and give you the upper hand in beating type 2 diabetes and achieving a healthy weight. Following are four blends we have found to be helpful. As a rule of thumb, you'll want to switch your protocol every three to four weeks for the best results.

NOTE
Use only one of these recipes at a time; in other words, don't take capsules at the same time you use a body oil or a roll-on.

BLOOD SUGAR-BALANCING BLEND (OPTION #1)

15 drops oregano essential oil

15 drops cinnamon bark essential oil

15 drops fenugreek essential oil

15 drops cumin essential oil

15 drops myrtle essential oil

BLOOD SUGAR-BALANCING BLEND (OPTION #2)

50 drops cinnamon bark essential oil

25 drops cumin essential oil

10 drops fenugreek essential oil

BLOOD SUGAR-BALANCING BLEND (OPTION #3)

50 drops melissa essential oil

25 drops lavender essential oil

10 drops geranium essential oil

BLOOD SUGAR-BALANCING BLEND (OPTION #4)

50 drops bergamot essential oil

20 drops peppermint essential oil

10 drops lavender essential oil

5 drops oregano essential oil

SUPPLIES

5-ml essential oil bottles

1. Mix the essential oils for each option in a 5-ml bottle.

2. Use as directed in the following recipes.

Blood Sugar-Balancing Roll-On

10 drops of one of the Blood Sugar-Balancing Blends (above)

Carrier oil of choice (fractionated coconut, jojoba, and sweet almond oils all work well)

SUPPLIES

10-ml glass roller bottle

1. Drop the essential-oil blend into the roller bottle.

2. Fill the bottle with the carrier oil. Shake vigorously for 10 seconds.

3. Apply over your abdomen and lower back twice a day.

NOTE

Test these blends first on the back of your hand or bottoms of your feet to ensure your body responds well to the blend. Immediately discontinue use if irritation occurs.

Blood Sugar–Balancing Body Oil

15 drops of one of the Blood Sugar–Balancing Blends (page 278)

1 ounce (6 teaspoons) carrier oil of choice (we use Mama Z's Oil Base, page 274, or fractionated coconut, jojoba, or sweet almond oil)

SUPPLIES
Small glass jar with a tight-fitting lid

1. Drop the essential-oil blend into the glass jar.

2. Add the carrier oil and mix.

3. Apply over your abdomen and lower back twice a day.

NOTE
First test this on the back of your hand or bottoms of your feet to make sure your body responds well to the blend. Discontinue use immediately if irritation occurs.

Blood Sugar–Balancing Capsule

3 drops of one of the Blood Sugar–Balancing Blends (page 278)

Raw coconut oil or extra-virgin olive oil

SUPPLIES
Pipette
Size 00 vegan gel capsule

1. Using a pipette, drop the essential-oil blend into the bottom half (the narrower one) of the capsule.

2. Use the pipette to fill the remaining space in the half capsule with coconut or extra-virgin olive oil.

3. Fit the wider top half of the capsule over the bottom half and secure it snugly.

4. Immediately swallow the capsule (see Note) with water on an empty stomach. Take twice daily.

NOTE
Do *not* make and store these capsules for future use.

HEAL GUT AND DIGESTIVE DISORDERS

Because of their rapid skin permeability and bioavailability, essential oils are adept at helping treat digestive and gut disorders. Cultures across the globe have traditionally enjoyed cardamom, ginger, fennel, and peppermint oils with great success. We have found that the following remedies work wonderfully.

Nausea-Soothing Diffuser Blend

2 drops ginger essential oil

2 drops lemon essential oil

2 drops peppermint essential oil

SUPPLIES
Diffuser

1. Fill the diffuser with water as directed in the manufacturer's instructions.

2. Add the ginger, lemon, and peppermint essential oils to the water.

3. Turn on the diffuser when you get an upset stomach or feel nauseated, sit by the diffuser, and relax for a few minutes. Be sure to take intentional slow, deep breaths.

4. Turn off the diffuser when the nausea or tummy upset goes away.

NOTE
You can keep this mixture in the diffuser and use it daily until it is empty.

Nausea-Soothing Inhaler

Store this in your purse so you can reach for it whenever you feel nauseated, and be sure to keep one handy at work.

7 drops cardamom essential oil

7 drops ginger essential oil

7 drops lemon essential oil

SUPPLIES
Precut organic cotton pad

Aromatherapy inhaler

Small glass bowl (optional)

Tweezers (optional)

1. Place a cotton pad in the inhaler tube.

2. Drop the cardamom, ginger, and lemon essential oils directly on the cotton pad. Alternatively, drop the essential oils in a glass bowl, rolling the cotton pad in the oils to absorb them. Then, using tweezers, insert the pad into the inhaler tube.

3. When you feel nauseated or as though you might vomit, open the inhaler and take a few deep breaths.

Nausea-Soothing Roll-On

4 drops ginger essential oil

2 drops lemon essential oil

2 drops peppermint essential oil

2 drops spearmint essential oil

Carrier oil of choice (fractionated coconut, jojoba, and sweet almond oils all work well)

SUPPLIES
10-ml glass roller bottle

1. Drop the ginger, lemon, peppermint, and spearmint essential oils into the roller bottle.

2. Fill up the bottle with the carrier oil. Shake vigorously for 10 seconds.

3. Apply over your abdomen (see Note, page 275) as needed.

Tummy Ache Roll-On

3 drops cardamom essential oil

2 drops fennel essential oil

2 drops ginger essential oil

1 drop thyme essential oil

1 drop clove essential oil

1 drop tarragon essential oil

Carrier oil of choice (fractionated coconut, jojoba, and sweet almond oils all work well)

SUPPLIES
10-ml glass roller bottle

1. Drop the essential oils into the roller bottle.

2. Fill up the bottle with the carrier oil. Shake vigorously for 10 seconds.

3. Apply over your abdomen (see Note, page 275) as needed.

Gut-Healing Capsule

This blend is useful for Crohn's, irritable bowel syndrome (IBS), and ulcerative colitis.

2 drops peppermint essential oil

1 drop ginger essential oil

Raw coconut oil or extra-virgin olive oil

SUPPLIES
Pipette

Size 00 enteric-coated capsule (not a gelatin capsule)

1. Using a pipette, drop the essential oils into the bottom half (the narrower one) of the capsule.

2. Use the pipette to fill the remaining space in the capsule with coconut or extra-virgin olive oil.

3. Fit the wider top half of the capsule over the bottom half and secure it snugly.

4. Immediately swallow the capsule with water on an empty stomach. Take twice daily.

NOTE
Do *not* make and store these capsules for future use.

Leaky Gut Capsule

2 drops oregano essential oil

Raw coconut oil or extra-virgin olive oil

SUPPLIES
Pipette

Size 00 enteric-coated capsule (not a gelatin capsule)

1. Using a pipette, drop the oregano essential oil into the bottom half (the narrower one) of the capsule.

2. Use the pipette to fill the remaining space in the capsule with coconut or extra-virgin olive oil.

3. Fit the wider top half over the bottom half of the capsule and secure it snugly.

4. Immediately swallow the capsule with water on an empty stomach. Take twice daily.

NOTE
Do *not* make and store these capsules for future use.

SOOTHE INFLAMMATION

In chapter 6, we discussed the most potent anti-inflammatory components in essential oils and which oils are best to soothe inflammation. Remember, when using these anti-inflammatory oils, you'll more than likely discover that certain blends work better for you than others, so be sure to refer back to chapter 6 for alternatives and different ideas.

Anti-inflammation Diffuser Blend

1 drop clove essential oil

1 drop copaiba essential oil

1 drop eucalyptus essential oil

1 drop orange essential oil

1 drop rosemary essential oil

SUPPLIES
Diffuser

1. Fill the diffuser with water as directed in the manufacturer's instructions.

2. Add the essential oils to the water.

3. Turn on the diffuser, sit down, and relax. Be sure to take intentional slow, deep breaths for a few minutes.

4. Turn off the diffuser when done.

NOTE
You can keep this mixture in the diffuser and use it daily until the diffuser is empty.

Anti-inflammation Inhaler

7 drops clove essential oil

7 drops eucalyptus essential oil

7 drops orange essential oil

SUPPLIES

Precut organic cotton pad

Aromatherapy inhaler

Small glass bowl (optional)

Tweezers (optional)

1. Place a cotton pad in the inhaler tube.

2. Drop the essential oils directly on the cotton pad. Alternatively, drop the essential oils into a glass bowl and roll the cotton pad in the oils to absorb them. Then, using tweezers, insert the pad into the inhaler tube.

3. Open the inhaler and take a few deep breaths throughout the day.

4. Store this in your purse so you can reach for it whenever you feel inflamed joints flare up or when you're stressed, as that triggers inflammation. Be sure to keep one handy at work.

Anti-inflammation Roll-On

4 drops ginger essential oil

2 drops lemon essential oil

2 drops peppermint essential oil

2 drops spearmint essential oil

Carrier oil of choice (fractionated coconut, jojoba, and sweet almond oil all work well)

SUPPLIES

10-ml glass roller bottle

1. Drop the essential oils into the roller bottle.

2. Fill up the bottle with the carrier oil. Shake vigorously for 10 seconds.

3. Apply over your abdomen (see Note, page 275) as needed.

Anti-inflammation Capsule

1 drop copaiba essential oil

1 drop orange essential oil

1 drop peppermint essential oil

Raw coconut oil or extra-virgin olive oil

SUPPLIES
Pipette

Size 00 vegan gel capsule

1. Using a pipette, drop the copaiba, orange, and peppermint essential oils into the bottom half (the narrower one) of the capsule.

2. Use the pipette to fill the remaining space in the half capsule with coconut or extra-virgin olive oil.

3. Fit the wider half of the capsule over the bottom half and secure it snugly.

4. Immediately swallow the capsule with water on an empty stomach. Take twice daily.

NOTE

Do *not* make and store these capsules for future use.

GET BETTER SLEEP AND REDUCE STRESS

When you think of reducing stress and achieving a peaceful, calm state, lavender essential oil immediately comes to mind. Using it can be as simple as adding a few drops of lavender to your diffuser, but if you need some extra support or are looking to spice it up, try the following healing remedies!

Better Sleep Diffuser Blend

2 drops lavender essential oil

2 drops Roman chamomile essential oil

2 drops vetiver essential oil

SUPPLIES
Diffuser

1. Fill the diffuser with water as directed in the manufacturer's instructions.

2. Add the essential oils to the water (see Note, page 276).

3. Turn on the diffuser 10 to 20 minutes before bedtime and set it to run throughout the night.

Citrus-Lover's Anxiety Inhaler

From The Healing Power of Essential Oils

5 drops orange essential oil

5 drops bergamot essential oil

5 drops sandalwood essential oil

5 drops ylang-ylang essential oil

SUPPLIES

Precut organic cotton pad

Aromatherapy inhaler

Small glass bowl (optional)

Tweezers (optional)

1. Place a cotton pad in the inhaler tube.

2. Drop the essential oils directly on the cotton pad.

3. Secure the cap and store the inhaler in your desk drawer, purse, or glove compartment so you always have it handy.

4. When a panic attack hits or you feel stressed, simply open the inhaler and take a few deep breaths of the vapor from the tube.

Better Sleep Inhaler

This remedy is designed for travelers, but it can also provide extra bedside support.

7 drops lavender essential oil

7 drops Roman chamomile essential oil

7 drops vetiver essential oil

SUPPLIES

Precut organic cotton pad

Aromatherapy inhaler

Small glass bowl (optional)

Tweezers (optional)

1. Place a cotton pad in the inhaler tube.

2. Drop the essential oils directly on the cotton pad. Alternatively, drop the essential oils into a glass bowl and roll the cotton pad in the oils to absorb them. Then, using tweezers, insert the pad into the inhaler tube.

3. Open the inhaler and take a few deep breaths before turning in.

Better Sleep Roll-On

4 drops lavender essential oil

4 drops Roman chamomile essential oil

4 drops vetiver essential oil

Carrier oil of choice (fractionated coconut, jojoba, and sweet almond oils all work well)

SUPPLIES

10-ml glass roller bottle

1. Drop the essential oils into the roller bottle.

2. Fill the bottle with the carrier oil. Shake vigorously for 10 seconds.

3. Massage into the back of your neck, your shoulders, and your feet (see Note, page 275) before bed.

Better Sleep Capsule

1 drop lavender essential oil

1 drop Roman chamomile essential oil

1 drop vetiver essential oil

Raw coconut oil or extra-virgin olive oil

SUPPLIES

Pipette

Size 00 vegan gel capsule

1. Thirty minutes before going to bed, using a pipette, drop the essential oils into the bottom half (the narrower one) of the capsule.

2. Use the pipette to fill the remaining space in the capsule with coconut or extra-virgin olive oil.

3. Fit the top half of the capsule over the bottom half and secure it snugly.

4. Immediately swallow the capsule (see Note) with water.

NOTE

Do *not* make and store these capsules for future use.

Restful Evening Detox Bath

From The Healing Power of Essential Oils

3 drops lavender essential oil

2 drops Roman chamomile essential oil

2 drops ylang-ylang essential oil

1 tablespoon jojoba oil

1 cup plain Epsom salts

¼ cup apple cider vinegar

SUPPLIES

Medium glass bowl

1. In a glass bowl, mix the essential oils and the jojoba oil.

2. Add the Epsom salts and cider vinegar and mix thoroughly.

3. Fill your bathtub with the warmest water you can stand, while slowly pouring the oils-and-salts mixture into the running water.

4. Soak your whole body (see Note) for 20 to 30 minutes.

5. To avoid feeling faint as you exit the bath, do it slowly: first sit up, then kneel, and finally stand.

NOTE

Test this first on the back of your hand or bottoms of your feet to make sure your body responds well to the blend. Discontinue use immediately if irritation occurs.

THE ESSENTIAL EXERCISE PROGRAM

Changing your diet without making any changes in your activity level is unlikely to achieve the transformative experience you are seeking. Sure, you'll lose some weight, but you'll never look and feel your best. Let's take it to the max! The Essential Exercise Program is Mama Z's take on high-intensity interval training, known as HIIT. With four kids, a business, a household to run, and her role as a group fitness instructor, she is well aware that time is of the essence.

What Is HIIT?

A big reason why exercise winds up at the bottom of many people's to-do list is the misconception that it requires an hour a day to get results. If this describes you, good news: Researchers at McMaster University have uncovered that just six minutes of intense "sprint" exercise a week could be as effective as an hour of daily moderate activity![1] We'd recommend going one step further and alternating this all-out sprint approach with cool-down recovery periods, during which you perform a less intense exercise, and limit your training sessions to just 15 to 20 minutes a day.

Think of this approach, also called burst training, as alternating sprints with walking instead of running a marathon. Cycles of intense exertion followed by slower recovery periods quickly burn fat and build muscle.

If you are just starting to exercise, trust us, you can commit to just 15 to 20 minutes a day. If exercise is already a part of your life, you are likely ready to ramp it up even more!

Less Fat in Less Time

The HIIT approach saves you time as an efficient fat burner, in large part thanks to its ability to manage the hormones primarily responsible for weight gain and eating, namely the following:

- *Ghrelin,* which moderates the release of the "hunger hormone," which stimulates the appetite, particularly for sweet, salty, and fried foods, and slows down fat usage.
- *Leptin,* the "starvation hormone," makes you feel full and manages long-term energy balance to help weight loss.
- *Growth hormone* is stimulated, thereby increasing lean body mass and reducing fat mass.

Substantial research shows ghrelin and growth hormone increase and leptin decreases after burst-training workouts, making HIIT one of the best ways to manage your hunger cues and stimulate your hormones to facilitate weight loss.[2]

Overall Improved Health

In addition to burning body fat and helping control hormonal cues that could undermine your best intention, HIIT also provides these benefits:

- Boosts cardiovascular health
- Improves muscle tone
- Helps define your abs
- Minimizes wrinkles and firms skin
- Increases energy level

- Boosts your metabolism even several hours after you finish your workout
- Improves libido

And, according to a 2012 presentation at the European Society of Cardiology, HIIT activates telomerase, an anti-aging enzyme, and reduces p53 expression, the most commonly mutated gene in people with cancer.[3] Wow!

What HIIT Teaches Your Body

Dr. Z here. The idea is that if the exercise is intense enough, the body winds up in "oxygen debt," and much-needed energy is thus pulled from the glycogen stored in the muscles. Once oxygen is restored to the body, it switches to pull energy from fat stores. In essence, HIIT teaches the body that muscles feed the body during exercise and fat feeds the body the rest of the time.

We advise that you exercise first thing in the morning to control your leptin, ghrelin, and growth hormone levels throughout the day. Exercising on an empty stomach has been shown to improve glucose tolerance and insulin sensitivity,[4] which helps improves weight loss, curbs cravings for unhealthy foods, and helps prevent type 2 diabetes.

One last caveat before we get to the exercises: Don't overdo it. You'll know that you've pushed yourself too hard when you experience dizziness, vertigo, nausea, or pain. You also may suffer from insomnia, chronic fatigue, delayed recovery time, elevated resting heart rate, and even a disinterest in exercise, which defeats the entire purpose of exercising in the first place!

And don't follow the adage "No pain, no gain." Nothing could be further from the truth. You'll know that you've pushed yourself too hard when you experience sharp and stabbing or dull and achy pain in your body. This is a sign of muscle, ligament, or tendon damage. General "soreness" is something altogether different and is completely normal for a day or two after working out.

Now over to Mama Z.

The Essential Workout

The program I've designed is similar to the one I use myself and as a group fitness instructor with students at all levels of fitness. As with everything else in the Essential Oils Diet, you get to design your own program. Following are three approaches you can take for your warm-up, which is *essential*—there's that word again—to warm up your muscles and reduce the risk of injury.

Then I'll introduce you to the moves that tone every major muscle group in your body, with emphasis on your abdominals. Strong abdominals allow you to hold your tummy in, among many other benefits, making you look slimmer and your clothes fit better. Don't be intimidated by the list that follows. If you're new to exercise or it has been a while, you can start with just some of the exercises and gradually increase your moves as you build your strength and endurance.

For almost every movement, I have provided modifications that allow you to make the basic exercises easier or, in a few cases, more challenging. Be sure to record your exercise activity in your Transformation Journal. I suspect you will be pleasantly surprised at how quickly you will see that increasing your commitment results in dramatic improvements in your energy level, endurance, muscle tone, and perhaps even your weight.

Use this week-by-week schedule to ramp up your workout as you increase your fitness levels.

To watch Mama Z demonstrate how to properly perform the exercises in this section, visit EssentialOilsDiet.com.

Weeks 1 and 2

Do tempo intervals three times per week. These are short, 10-second all-out bursts done at a moderate-to-intense pace, with 50 seconds of slow activity done as the "rest." Speed walk, jog, bike, or do jumping jacks or whatever type of exercise you like. Try not to overcomplicate things. Perform a total of 10 intervals.

- *Warm-up:* Spend some time loosening up your muscles and get your head in the game by following the Essential Eight Warm-Up on page 295.
- *Burst:* 10 seconds at a max effort level of 5 out of 10.
- *Recovery:* 50 seconds of easy exercise at a minimal effort level of 2 out of 10.
- *Number of intervals:* 10

Weeks 3 and 4

Take what you've been doing during weeks 1 and 2 and kick it up a notch. Try different exercises than what you've been doing and focus on a total-body workout, exercising multiple muscle groups and body parts.

- *Warm-up:* Spend some time loosening up your muscles and get your head in the game by following the Essential Eight Warm-Up on page 295.
- *Burst:* 30 seconds at a max effort level of 7 out of 10.
- *Recovery:* 60 seconds of easy-to-moderate exercise at an effort level of 5 out of 10.
- *Number of intervals:* 10

Week 5 and Beyond

Ramp up to a four- or five-day weekly workout regimen and start to implement all of the exercises in the Essential Workout on page 297. Choose three or four exercises each day.

- *Warm-up:* Spend some time loosening up your muscles and get your head in the game by following the Essential Eight Warm-Up on page 295.
- *Burst:* 30 seconds at a max effort level of 7 out of 10.
- *Recovery:* 60 seconds of easy-to-moderate exercise at an effort level of 5 out of 10.
- *Number of intervals:* 10

A Minimum of Gear

If you don't belong to a health club and will be working out at home, you may need to make a small investment in exercise gear. A yoga or Pilates mat is handy, but a folded blanket is a no-cost stand-in. An exercise ball will set you back about $8; be sure to get the correct size for your height. A set of weights starts at about $5, or use quart-size plastic milk containers filled with sand or water; the handles make them super easy to grip. A double ab wheel costs well under $10. Also, having a five-foot broom handle will come in handy, especially for abs. Having a few different medicine balls of varying weight will be useful; two-pound and five-pound medicine balls are recommended to get started. Walmart and Amazon are great resources; be sure to do some price comparisons among manufacturers. Gold's Gym products are particularly well priced.

Now let's get moving!

The Essential Eight Warm-Up

An active warm-up, rather than static stretches, loosens up the muscles you will be using in the strength-building, fat-burning workout itself.

Personalize your warm-up: Spend 5 to 10 minutes going up and down stairs, walking briskly, or following my martial arts warm-up below.

Do 16 to 20 reps on each side for each of these warm-up exercises:

1. *Front Kicks:* Raise your right knee to a 90-degree angle, then kick straight forward. Lower. Repeat with your left leg.

2. *Roundhouse Kicks:* Begin by taking a 45-degree step with your left leg, opening up your hips. Bring your right knee up and across the front of your body. Turn your hips over and extend your right leg in a "kicking" motion. Bring your right leg back to the starting position. Repeat with your left leg.

3. *Side Kicks:* Kick to the right side of your body, lifting your knee up and pointing your bottom to the direction you are kicking as you extend your heel out to the side. Your toes should be neutral or pointed down. Repeat with your left leg to the left side of your body.

4. *Standing Front Leg Lifts:* Stand with your legs shoulder-width apart. Extend your right leg straight up as far as you can, stretching your hamstrings with your toes pointed toward the ceiling. Repeat with your left leg. You should feel like you're walking in place like a toy soldier.

5. *Standing Side Leg Lifts:* Stand with your legs shoulder-width apart. Extend your right leg out to the side 90 degrees, stretching your hips with your toes pointed toward the ceiling. Repeat with your left leg. After 16 to 20 reps, repeat the motion with your toes pointed forward, not up to the ceiling.

6. *Back Hip Flexors:* Stand, supporting yourself, if necessary, beside a wall or a sturdy chair, and lift your right leg back and up with your toes pointed, relaxing your hips as you do the stretch. Repeat with your left leg.

7. *Arm Circles:* Stand, raise both of your arms to your side at shoulder height, and rotate forward in a tight to increasingly wide circle. Repeat, rotating backward.
8. *Washing Machine:* With your arms raised to chest level and your elbows bent at a 45-degree angle, twist your torso from left to right and let your arms swing; repeat from right to left.

Personalize Your Program

I've divided the exercises into three categories: abdominals, upper body, and lower body. Here's how you can design your own program:

- *Modify the moves.* I'll explain how to make most of the moves easier or more challenging to suit your level of fitness and then modify them as you get stronger.
- *Decide how many sets.* I've recommended the number of sets (or in one case, the elapsed time), but you can do fewer sets if you wish.
- *Decide how many reps.* Again, I've recommended a minimum number, but you can do fewer if necessary.
- *Choose how many exercises to do in one session.* My strong recommendation is to do all the exercises in a single group rather than cherry-pick among them, as the order is designed to coordinate with the HIIT concept of interspersing more vigorous moves with those that require less exertion.
- *Decide which body parts to focus on.* If you are a seasoned exerciser, you might run through the entire list of exercises after your warm-up, or you can choose to focus on abs one day, upper body the next, then lower body. Or focus on abs and upper body one day, and abs and lower body the following day. My preference would be to always do the ab exercises first, if you can manage that.

If you are going to do just a couple of exercises to start, do the Arm Circles (page 300) and Mountain Climbers (below), but always be sure to do the warm-up exercises (page 295) first.

In addition to the instructions below, you can watch me perform each exercise in a video tutorial at EssentialOilsDiet.com. Time to move!

The Essential Workout

LOWER-BODY MOVES

MOUNTAIN CLIMBERS

How to do it: Assume a plank position (also known as a push-up position) with your hands spread wide on the ground and your body and neck in a neutral position. Alternate moving your right and left legs forward as though you are running. Keep your hips low and contract your core.

TIME: 1 MINUTE

Modification: Spread your hands on a step of a staircase instead of the floor for greater support.

STRAIGHT-ARM JUMPING JACKS

How to do it: Raise your arms, keeping them as straight as possible, over your head, touching when they meet and returning them to your sides, as you simultaneously jump up and down, opening your legs wide and then closing them in sync with your arms.

2 OR 3 SETS; 35 TO 50 REPS PER SET

Modifications: Move your arms as above, but don't move your legs as wide apart; walk your legs out instead of jumping; or simply do the arm motions with no leg motion.

FORWARD LUNGES

How to do it: Step forward with your right leg and drop your left knee as close to the floor as you can while placing your hands on your hips. Don't let your right knee go beyond your toes when lunging. Return to the starting position. Repeat with your left leg.

30 REPS PER SIDE

Modifications: Don't dip your knee all the way to the ground. Or hold on to a chair as you step and lunge.

SPEED SKATING (SIDE LUNGES)

How to do it: Push off to one side, pressing your hip out and bending your knee, while simultaneously straightening your opposite leg and dipping your opposite arm as though you are ice-skating or roller-skating, then pushing off to the other side while placing your hands on your hips.

60 REPS IN TOTAL IN ONE CONTINUOUS MOVEMENT (30 PER SIDE)

Modifications: Don't dip your knee down as far. Or hold on to a chair as you step and lunge.

STEP-BACK LUNGES

How to do it: Stand up straight with your legs shoulder-width apart. Take a large step backward with your right leg and lower your hips so that your left thigh is parallel to the floor and your left knee is in line with your ankle. Try to get your right knee as close to the floor as possible while placing your hands on your hips. Make sure your left knee doesn't go over your toes when lunging. Return to the starting position. Repeat with your left leg.

30 REPS PER SIDE

Modifications: Don't drop your knee as close to the ground. Or hold on to a chair as you step and lunge. Or do a static lunge by going up and down on your knee without moving backward and forward.

SQUATS

How to do it: With your feet shoulder-width apart, slowly bend your knees to set your bottom back as though you are sitting on a chair while placing your hands at your waist or clasping them together at chest level. Keep your chest up and look up at the ceiling. Then press through your heels as you come up to starting position, moving only the legs. Make sure that your knees never go over your toes.

30 REPS

Modifications: Don't dip down as far. Or hold on to the back of a chair as you sit back to support youself.

FIRE HYDRANTS

How to do it: Get on your hands and knees on an exercise mat or folded blanket, with your wrists directly under your shoulders and your knees in line with your hips. Lift your right knee up and out to the side, making sure that your knee is level with the rest of the leg. Repeat with your left leg.

30 REPS EACH LEG

MULE AND ROUND KICKS

How to do it: Get on your hands and knees on an exercise mat or folded blanket, with your wrists directly under your shoulders and your knees in line with your hips. Pull your navel toward your back. Lift your right leg directly behind you (like a mule kicking), keeping your back flat and maintaining a 90-degree angle in your knees with your foot flexed. Repeat, chambering your leg between each kick, without putting it down. After completing the reps on your right side, point your knee to the front, maintaining a 90-degree angle, and kick directly out in front of you, completing the same number of reps. Repeat both kicks with your left leg.

30 REPS EACH LEG FOR BOTH KICKS

UPPER-BODY MOVES

NEGATIVE PUSH-UPS

How to do it: Assume a plank position (also known as a push-up position) with your arms bent and parallel to your body with your forearms on the floor so your body makes a straight line from your heels to your shoulders. In a downward motion, bend your elbows tight in to the body, lower your body slowly to a count of 5, letting your chest touch the ground first. Then push back on to your knees and back up to plank position.

2 OR 3 SETS; 15 REPS PER SET

Modifications: Do negative push-ups on walls, stairs, or on your knees. Or do regular push-ups from the floor. Do all to a count of 5 while holding your elbows tight to your body.

ARM CIRCLES AND HAND GRIP EXERCISES

How to do it: With your arms straight and extended out to each side at shoulder level, make tight forward and then backward circles. Next move your arms in front of you at the same height and open your fingers as far apart as possible, fully extending each finger. Then close your fists and repeat. Once you do this with your hands in front of you for 15 seconds, move your hands over your head and continue the open and close motion for 15 seconds. Next extend your hands to either side of your body and continue the open and close motion for another 15 seconds. Finally, return your hands to the front of your body and repeat for the last 15 seconds.

ARM CIRCLES: 1 MINUTE FORWARD, 1 MINUTE BACKWARD

GRIP EXERCISE: 1 MINUTE

Modification: Don't raise your arms up all the way to the side.

REACH FOR HEAVEN

How to do it: Standing tall and straight, lift your arms over your head and touch the tops of your hands together. Bring your arms down in front of your body 90 degrees and bend over as far as you can (trying to touch your toes) without feeling pain, while keeping your legs straight, but without locking your knees. Repeat.

35 REPS

ABDOMINALS

AB WHEEL ROLLOUT

How to do it: Using a double ab wheel for extra strength and support and with your knees on an exercise mat or folded blanket, kneel and round your back to start the exercise. Roll out your arms in front of you as far as you can, then roll back to the starting position. Repeat. Set a goal for how low you can go and push yourself a little farther each time. Always keep your back straight; do not arch your back or let your abdomen sag. Eventually, you want your back to be as flat as possible.

15 TO 50 REPS

Modification: Don't go down as far.

STAR CRUNCHES

How to do it: Lie on your back, with your arms and legs spread out and holding a light to medium weight in each hand. Your arms and your legs should not be touching the ground. Bring your arms and knees together in one motion so your elbows and knees touch (meeting over your waist), crunching your abdomen and almost rolling into a ball. (If you have no weights, use cans from your pantry.) Return to the starting position. Repeat.

25 TO 50 REPS

Modification: Do without weights.

EXERCISE BALL CRUNCHES

How to do it: Sit on an exercise ball with your knees at a 90-degree angle, then walk your legs out, pressing your lower back into the ball and rolling your belly button up so it is facing the ceiling. Place your arms behind your head to lightly support it (but don't tug on your neck). If this is difficult, fold them on your chest. As you do your reps, exhale as you crunch and inhale as you lower, starting with regular crunches, then progressing to crunches on the right side and the left side, alternating if you prefer. Finally do regular crunches holding a 3- to 5-pound medicine ball at your chest, working your way up to a heavier ball.

25 TO 50 REPS FOR EACH OF THE FOUR CRUNCH VARIATIONS

Modifications: No medicine ball? Just do the last set of crunches on the exercise ball. Or omit the right and left side crunches if you have diastasis recti; instead, do more regular crunches on the exercise ball. Your total reps should be between 100 and 200.

EXERCISE BALL EXTENSIONS

How to do it: Press your lower back into the ball and roll your belly button up so it is facing the ceiling. Place your hands one on top of another, reach them back toward the wall behind you, and pulse. Start with reps of regular pulses, followed by reps to the right and then to the left (or alternate between right and left). Then do reps of regular pulses holding a 3- to 5-pound medicine ball to start, working your way up to a heavier ball.

25 TO 50 REPS FOR EACH OF THE FOUR CRUNCH VARIATIONS

Modifications: No medicine ball? Just do an additional set of regular pulses on the exercise ball. Omit the right and left side if you have diastasis recti; instead, do more regular crunches on the exercise ball. Your total reps should be between 100 and 200.

BROOMSTICK AB TWISTS

How to do it: Place a broomstick or a stick attachment for a paint roller behind your neck with your arms extended out on either side and your hands holding the stick. Twist right and then left for 25 reps, then lean back and twist for another 25 reps, then lean forward and twist for another 25 reps. Slowly work your way up to standing for 25 reps. Finally, do another 25 straight standing reps.

25 TO 50 REPS EACH OF FIVE WAYS

SUPERMAN

How to do it: Lying on an exercise mat or blanket on your stomach, reach your arms straight out in front of you as if you were trying to fly. Reach as far as you can forward, lifting your hands and feet off the ground. Hold them for a split second at the top as you lift up, then return to your resting position.

25 TO 50 REPS

Modification: For greater intensity, put 3- to 5-pound weights on your ankles and wrists.

NOTE
If you cannot do any of the abdominal exercises or modifications above, do the following.

NINJA TURTLES

How to do it: Lie on your back on the floor with your hands behind your head, bend your knees and lift your knees up to your chest so your heels are by your buttocks, twist right and left on your back as though you are a turtle stuck upside down on your shell. For a greater challenge, touch your heels with the corresponding hand and twist right and left.

50 TO 100 REPS

Again, you can watch Mama Z demonstrate how to perform these exercises at EssentialOilDiet.com.

ACKNOWLEDGMENTS

From both of us:

Our sincere love and heartfelt gratitude to God, and to all of the behind-the-scenes people He put in our path who helped make this book a reality.

To Mom and Dad Frawley, yay, we did it! You supported us to chase our dreams, and look what happened! Without you, our global Bible health ministry would not exist and this book would never have been written. We are also eternally grateful for everything that you have taught us about business and work ethics, and for inspiring us to never settle for anything but God's best in our lives.

To Papa Enoch, your ministry has inspired thousands to live for Christ and to seek the abundant life through many of the principles shared in this book. Through your mentorship, you helped lay the foundation for much of what is written in these pages, and we are grateful for the time that you spent teaching us these eternal truths.

To Miss Alex Chapman, Miss Natalie, and Miss Faye, for helping with the kiddos during those long hours and for being Mama Z's right-hand gals during her cooking class videos. We all love you!

To Shana Lee, for being true to whom God called you to be. You are an amazing soul frequency coach, and we so appreciate your wisdom and sage advice when we need it most. Your love and encouragement have helped transform us into who we are today.

To Jason and Loren, Gabe and Brittany, Brandon and Brittany, Chris and Jessica, Aaron and Krupa, Victor, Daniel, Craig, Joel, Beth, and the entire crew, you are all so precious to us, and we will be forever grateful that you have welcomed us into your "Fit Fam" with open arms. Thank you for your friendship, for your love, and for your support as we all strive to be healthy in spirit, soul, and body!

To Reggie and Amy Black, K.C. and Monica Craichy, Stephen and Amy Ezell, Ty and Charlene Bollinger, Chris and Micah Wark, Michael and Lillian Tyrrell, Dr. Tony and Marcy Jiminez, Jonathan and Lori Otto, Jill Winger, Dr. Peter Osborne, Dr. Brian Mowll, and Robyn Openshaw, your ministries have meant so much to us and to the world. It is an honor to call you friends and colleagues.

To Pastor Barclay, the wisdom you have shared in your preaching is sprinkled throughout this book and has forever marked how we live and journey through life together.

To Whit, Elizabeth, Angela, Erica, Carrie, Krystal, Jendi, Susan, John, Christa, Trish, Tamika, Victoria, Sher, Dee, Matthew, Chris, and the entire NaturalLivingFamily.com team, your hard work and determination have been priceless! Thank you so much for all that you do to make NaturalLivingFamily.com the number one most-visited website devoted to biblical health on the planet!

To Olivia Bell Buehl, for your brilliant insight and savvy wordsmithing. Your help putting together this manuscript was absolutely priceless. You are a gem, and it has been an honor to work with you on this project.

To our literary agents, John Maas and Celeste Fine Folch, for your advocacy, hard work, and for being our trusted guides. You are the best!

To the wonderful team at Harmony Books: Alyse Diamond, Christina Foxley, Danielle Curtis, Tammy Blake, Connie Capone, and the unsung heroes in the fact-checking and copyediting departments—all we can say is "Wow!" You are the dream team, and we couldn't have asked for a better group of professionals to make all of this happen.

Last, but not least, to all of our members, newsletter subscribers, and social media followers, for your thought-provoking questions, kind comments, and unending support. You are the reason we do what we do, and we thank you for helping spread this message to millions of people across the globe!

. . .

From Mama Z:

To Yvonne Rundell, one of my closest friends who is now in Heaven with our Heavenly Father, I am so thankful for your foresight, friendship, and encouragement that helped birth this book. Your passion ignited the fire within me to get these recipes and healthy natural living tips in the hands of so many. I love you, my dear sister in Christ, and I will always be grateful for the time we had together. I dedicate this book to you and your memory.

To Mary Ellen Miller, you have always been my biggest cheerleader. I've been blessed by your love and encouragement in more ways than you'll ever know. You have also been an amazing example of how a woman can succeed in both business and family, and you have taught me countless invaluable lessons. Your wisdom and love have helped shape me into the person that I am today.

To Lisa Miner, my best girlie friend, thank you for always encouraging me to be me, and for inspiring me to excellence. Your encouragement, love, and support have fueled me to be my best. Zero balance!

To Gayle and Lisa O, my Georgia Peaches! I love you girls and appreciate all of the hours of love and time we spent together during pageant. You make me feel my best and encourage me to strive to new heights!

To Sally Hecox, my lifelong friend, pageant coach, and director, I'm grateful for all the life lessons you have taught me over the years. You have helped me learn to never settle for anything less than my best in every area of my life.

To LaLona Richards, my pageant coach, you are like a sister to me. You have strengthened me and have held me accountable to be a well-rounded Proverbs 31 woman. With your help, I have competed at the highest level possible. I am so thankful for all of your encouragement, inspiration, and support.

To Leonora, Sandi, and Mrs. Buck, my mothers in the faith, without the countless hours you have spent sowing into my life and encouraging me with Godly principles, I would not be the person I am today.

NOTES

Preface: Meet the Elephants in the Room

1. "Adult Obesity Facts," Centers for Disease Control and Prevention, accessed August 7, 2018, https://www.cdc.gov/obesity/data/adult.html.

2. "Nutrition and Weight Management," Boston Medical Center, accessed August 7, 2018, https://www.bmc.org/nutrition-and-weight-management/weight-management.

3. "What Is Metabolic Syndrome?" American Heart Association, accessed August 24, 2018, https://www.heart.org/-/media/data-import/downloadables/pe-abh-what-is-metabolic-syndrome-ucm_300322.pdf.

4. S. Jay Olshansky, Douglas J. Passaro, Ronald C. Hershow, et al., "A Potential Decline in Life Expectancy in the United States in the 21st Century," *New England Journal of Medicine* 352, no. 11 (March 2005): 1138–45, https://doi.org/10.1056/NEJMsr043743.

Introduction: How Did We Get into This Mess?

1. Kelly M. Adams, W. Scott Butsch, and Martin Kohlmeier, "The State of Nutrition Education at US Medical Schools," *Journal of Biomedical Education* 2015, article ID 357627 (2015), http://dx.doi.org/10.1155/2015/357627.

2. "Adult Obesity Facts," Centers for Disease Control and Prevention, accessed August 24, 2018, https://www.cdc.gov/obesity/data/adult.html.

3. "Children and Adolescent Obesity Facts," Centers for Disease Control and Prevention, accessed August 7, 2018, https://www.cdc.gov/obesity/data/childhood.html.

4. "Obesity and Overweight," World Health Organization, accessed August 7, 2018, http://www.who.int/news-room/fact-sheets/detail/obesity-and-overweight.

Chapter 1: Why "Diets" Fail but Transformation Works

1. "National Obesity Rates & Trends," *State of Obesity,* Robert Wood Johnson Foundation, accessed August 28, 2018, https://stateofobesity.org/obesity-rates-trends-overview.

2. J. H. Ellenbroek, L. van Dijck, H. A. Töns, et al., "Long-Term Ketogenic Diet Causes Glucose Intolerance and Reduced β- and α-Cell Mass but No Weight Loss in Mice,"

American Journal of Physiology: Endocrinology and Metabolism 306, no. 5 (March 1, 2014): E552–58.

3. N. Douris, T. Melman, J. M. Pecherer, et al., "Adaptive Changes in Amino Acid Metabolism Permit Normal Longevity in Mice Consuming a Low-Carbohydrate Ketogenic Diet," *Biochimica et Biophysica Acta* 1852, 10 pt. A (October 2015): 2056–65.

4. "Metabolism and Weight Loss: How You Burn Calories," Mayo Clinic, accessed August 7, 2018, https://www.mayoclinic.org/healthy-lifestyle/weight-loss/in-depth/metabolism/art-20046508.

5. "Healthy Weight: How Can I Speed Up My Metabolism?" National Health Services, accessed August 9, 2018, https://www.nhs.uk/live-well/healthy-weight/metabolism-and-weight-loss.

6. M. Lenoir, F. Serre, L. Cantin, et al., "Intense Sweetness Surpasses Cocaine Reward," *PLOS ONE* 2, no. 8 (August 1, 2007): e698, https://doi.org/10.1371/journal.pone.0000698.

7. Gina Cleo, Paul Glasziou, Elaine Beller, et al., "Habit-Based Interventions for Weight Loss Maintenance in Adults with Overweight and Obesity: A Randomized Controlled Trial," *International Journal of Obesity* (April 23, 2018), https://doi.org/10.1038/s41366-018-0067-4.

8. P. Lally, C. H. M. van Jaarsveld, H. W. W. Potts, et al., "How Are Habits Formed: Modelling Habit Formation in the Real World," *European Journal of Social Psychology* 40, no. 6 (October 2010): 998–1009, https://doi.org/10.1002/ejsp.674.

Chapter 2: The Antidote to Chemical Soup: Bioactive-Rich Foods and Essential Oils

1. J.-H. Li, Z.-H. Wang, X.-J. Zhu, et al., "Health Effects from Swimming Training in Chlorinated Pools and the Corresponding Metabolic Stress Pathways," *PLoS ONE* 10, no. 3 (March 2015): e0119241, https://doi.org/10.1371/journal.pone.0119241.

2. J. Vlaanderen, K. von Veldhoven, L. Font-Ribera, et al., "Acute Changes in Serum Immune Markers due to Swimming in a Chlorinated Pool," *Environment International* 107 (August 2017): 1–11, https://doi.org/10.1016/j.envint.2017.04.009.

3. R. G. Wones and C. J. Glueck, "Effects of Chlorinated Drinking Water on Human Lipid Metabolism," *Environmental Health Perspectives* 69 (1986): 255–58.

4. V. Bougault and L.-P. Boulet, "Airways Disorders and the Swimming Pool," *Immunology and Allergy Clinics of North America* 33, no. 3 (August 2013): 395–408, https://doi.org/10.1016/j.iac.2013.02.008.

5. Greater Boston Physicians for Social Responsibility, *In Harm's Way: Toxic Threats to Child Development* (Cambridge, MA: GBPSR, 2000), accessed August 16, 2018, http://action.psr.org/site/DocServer/ihwcomplete.pdf?docID=5131.

6. J. McCandless, *Children with Starving Brains: A Medical Treatment Guide for Autism Spectrum Disorder,* 2nd ed. (Putney, VT: Bramble Books, 2003).

7. G. Vighi, F. Marcucci, L. Sense, et al., "Allergy and the Gastrointestinal System," *Clinical and Experimental Immunology* 153, suppl. 1 (September 2008): 3–6, https://doi.org/10.1111/j.1365-2249.2008.03713.x.

8. "11 Scary Statistics on Antibiotic Resistance," HealthResearchFunding.org, accessed August 7, 2018, https://healthresearchfunding.org/11-scary-statistics-on-antibiotic-resistance.

9. Ibid.

10. Ibid.

11. M. C. Noverr, R. M. Noggle, G. B. Toews, et al., "Role of Antibiotics and Fungal Microbiota in Driving Pulmonary Allergic Responses," *Infection and Immunity* 72, no. 9 (September 2004): 4996–5003, https://doi.org/10.1128/IAI.72.9.4996-5003.2004.

12. J. Brody, "Popular Antibiotics May Carry Serious Side Effects," *New York Times*, September 10, 2012, https://well.blogs.nytimes.com/2012/09/10/popular-antibiotics-may-carry-serious-side-effects/?ref=janeebrody.

13. J. S. Cohen, "Peripheral Neuropathy Associated with Fluoroquinolone," *Annals of Pharmacotherapy* 35, no. 12 (2001): 1540–47, https://doi.org/10.1345/aph.1Z429.

14. A. Béjaoui, H. Chaabane, M. Jemli, et al., "Essential Oil Composition and Antibacterial Activity of *Origanum vulgare* subsp. *glandulosum* Desf. at Different Phenological Stages," *Journal of Medicinal Food* 16, no. 12 (December 13, 2013): 1115–20, https://doi.org/10.1089/jmf.2013.0079.

15. "Bioactive Compound," ScienceDirect, accessed August 7, 2018, https://www.sciencedirect.com/topics/agricultural-and-biological-sciences/bioactive-compound.

16. Ibid.

17. H. K. Biesalski, J. W. Erdman, J. Hatchcock, et al., "Nutrient Reference Values for Bioactives: New Approaches Needed? A Conference Report," *European Journal of Nutrition* 52, suppl. 1 (April 2013): 1–9, https://doi.org/10.1007/s00394-013-0503-0.

18. Y. Wang, X. Miao, J. Sun, et al., "Oxidative Stress in Diabetes: Molecular Basis for Diet Supplementation," in *Molecular Nutrition and Diabetes* D. Mauricio, ed. (Boston: Academic Press, 2016), 65–72, https://doi.org/10.1016/B978-0-12-801585-8.00006-3.

19. P. M. Kris-Etherton, K. D. Hecker, A. Bonanome, et al., "Bioactive Compounds in Foods: Their Role in the Prevention of Cardiovascular Disease and Cancer," *American Journal of Medicine* 113, no. 9, suppl. 2 (December 30, 2002): 71–88, https://doi.org/10.1016/S0002-9343(01)00995-0.

20. D. A. Quintana Pacheco, D. Sookthai, C. Wittenbecher, et al., "Red Meat Consumption and Risk of Cardiovascular Diseases: Is Increased Iron Load a Possible Link?" *American Journal of Clinical Nutrition* 107, no. 1 (January 1, 2018): 113–19, https://doi.org/10.1093/ajcn/nqx014.

21. H. K. Biesalski, J. W. Erdman, J. Hatchcock. et al., "Nutrient Reference Values for Bioactives: New Approaches Needed? A Conference Report," *European Journal of Nutrition* 52, suppl. 1 (April 2013): 1–9, https://doi.org/10.1007/s00394-013-0503-0.

22. N. Mahfoudhi, R. Ksouri, and S. Hamdi, "Nanoemulsions as Potential Delivery Systems for Bioactive Compounds in Food Systems: Preparation, Characterization, and Applications in Food Industry," in *Emulsions: Nanotechnology in the Agri-Food Industry,* vol. 3, *Nanotechnology in the Agri-Food Industry* (Boston: Academic Press, 2016), 365–403, https://doi.org/10.1016/B978-0-12-804306-6.00011-8.

23. "Essential Oil," Encyclopedia Britannica, accessed August 9, 2018, https://www.britannica.com/topic/essential-oil.

24. N. Mahfoudhi, R. Ksouri, and S. Hamdi, "Nanoemulsions as Potential Delivery Systems for Bioactive Compounds in Food Systems: Preparation, Characterization, and Applications in Food Industry," in *Emulsions: Nanotechnology in the Agri-Food Industry,* vol. 3, *Nanotechnology in the Agri-Food Industry* (Boston: Academic Press, 2016), 365–403.

25. W. Jäger, G. Buchbauer, L. Jirovet, et al., "Percutaneous Absorption of Lavender Oil from a Massage Oil," *Journal of the Society of Cosmetic Chemists* 43, no. 1 (January/February 1992): 49–54.

26. R. Tisserand and R. Young, *Essential Oil Safety,* 2nd ed. (London: Churchill Livingstone Elsevier, 2014), 85–87.

Chapter 3: It's Not Your Fault: You've Been Misinformed

1. B. T. Hunter, "The Downside of Soybean Consumption," *Nutrition Digest* 38, no. 2, accessed October 21, 2018, http://americannutritionassociation.org/newsletter/downside-soybean-consumption-0.

2. Ibid.

3. G. E. Séralini, R. Mesnage, E. Claire, et al., "Genetically Modified Crops Safety Assessments: Present Limits and Possible Improvements," *Environmental Sciences Europe* 23, no. 10 (December 2011), https://doi.org/10.1186/2190-4715-23-10.

4. "Soy," WebMD, accessed August 4, 2018, https://www.webmd.com/vitamins/ai/ingredientmono-975/soy.

5. Kim Cross, "The Grass-Fed vs. Grain-Fed Beef Debate," *Cooking Light*, March 29, 2011, http://www.cnn.com/2011/HEALTH/03/29/grass.grain.beef.cookinglight.

6. "First-Ever US Tests of Farmed Salmon Show High Levels of Cancer-Causing PCBs," Environmental Working Group, accessed June 1, 2018, https://www.ewg.org/news/news-releases/2003/07/30/first-ever-us-tests-farmed-salmon-show-high-levels-cancer-causing-pcbs#.WxGSSFMvx-U.

7. "PCBs in Farmed Salmon: Test Results Show High Levels of Contamination," Environmental Working Group, July 30, 2003, https://www.ewg.org/research/pcbs-farmed-salmon#.W2T97i3MzOQ.

8. N. Burca and R. R. Watson, "Fish Oil Supplements, Contaminants, and Excessive Doses," in *Omega-3 Fatty Acids in Brain and Neurological Health,* R. R. Watson, ed. (Boston: Academic Press. 2014), 447–54, www.sciencedirect.com/science/article/pii/B9780124105270000363.

9. M. Rose, "Hazardous Chemicals as Animal Feed Contaminants and Methods for Their Detection," in *Animal Feed Contamination: Effects on Livestock and Food Safety,* J. Fink-Gremmels, ed. (Cambridge, UK: Woodhead Publishing, 2012), 117–30, https://www.sciencedirect.com/science/article/pii/B9781845697259500078.

10. A. Molassiotis and P. Peat, "Surviving Against All Odds: Analysis of 6 Case Studies of Patients with Cancer Who Followed the Gerson Therapy," *Integrative Cancer Therapies* 6, no. 1 (March 1, 2007): 80–88, https://doi.org/10.1177/1534735406298258.

11. H. J. Beckie, K. N. Harker, A. Légère, et al., "GM Canola: The Canadian Experience," *Farm Policy Journal* 8, no. 1 (Autumn 2011): 43–49, https://www.canolawatch.org/wpcontent/uploads/2011/10/20110309_FPJ_Aut11_Beckie.et_.al_.pdf.

12. H. Bartsch, J. Nair, R. W. Owen, "Dietary Polyunsaturated Fatty Acids and Cancers of the Breast and Colorectum: Emerging Evidence for Their Role as Risk Modifiers," *Carcinogenesis* 20, no. 12 (December 1, 1999): 2209–18, https://doi.org/10.1093/carcin/20.12.2209.

13. "Steps in Oil and Meal Processing," Canola Council of Canada, accessed August 4, 2018, https://www.canolacouncil.org/oil-and-meal/what-is-canola/how-canola-is-processed/steps-in-oil-and-meal-processing#SolventExtraction.

14. K. Gunnars, "Canola Oil: Good or Bad?" Healthline, March 9, 2014, https://www .healthline.com/nutrition/canola-oil-good-or-bad.

15. S. Fallon and M. G. Enig, "The Great Con-ola," Weston A. Price Foundation, July 28, 2002, https://www.westonaprice.org/health-topics/know-your-fats/the -great-con-ola.

16. S. O'Keefe, S. Gaskins-Wright, V. Wiley, et al., "Levels of *Trans* Geometrical Isomers of Essential Fatty Acids in Some Unhydrogenated U.S. Vegetable Oils," *Journal of Food Lipids* 1, no. 3 (September 1994): 165–76, https://doi.org/10.1111/j.1745-4522.1994 .tb00244.x.

17. S. A. Fallon and M. G. Enig, "The Oiling of America," extract from *Nexus* 6, no. 1 (December 1998–January 1999), accessed August 4, 2018, https://pdfs.semanticscholar .org/c929/ad22d48819170127597d26a5e70c38a49021.pdf.

18. K. Kavanagh, K. L. Jones, J. Sawyer, et al., "Trans Fat Diet Induces Abdominal Obesity and Changes in Insulin Sensitivity in Monkeys," *Obesity* 15, no. 7 (July 2007): 1675–84.

19. A. K. Thompson, A. M. Minihane, and C. M. Williams, "*Trans* Fatty Acids and Weight Gain," *International Journal of Obesity* 35 (2011): 315–24, https://doi.org/10.1038/ ijo.2010.141.

20. L. Mínguez-Alarcón, J. E. Chavarro, J. Mendiola, et al. "Fatty Acid Intake in Relation to Reproductive Hormones and Testicular Volume Among Young Healthy Men," *Asian Journal of Andrology* 19, no. 2 (2017): 184–90, https://doi.org/10.4103/1008-682X.190323.

21. E. Ginter and V. Simko, "New Data on Harmful Effects of Trans-Fatty Acids," *Bratislava Medical Journal* 117, no. 5 (2016): 251–53.

22. M. Dhibi, F. Brahmi, A. Mnari, et al., "The Intake of High Fat Diet with Different *Trans* Fatty Acid Levels Differentially Induces Oxidative Stress and Non-alcoholic Fatty Liver Disease (NAFLD) in Rats," *Nutrition & Metabolism* 8, no. 65 (2011), https://doi .org/10.1186/1743-7075-8-65.

23. S. Fallon and M. G. Enig, "The Great Con-ola," Weston A. Price Foundation, July 28, 2002, accessed August 4, 2018, https://www.westonaprice.org/health-topics/ know-your-fats/the-great-con-ola.

24. K. Zeratsky, "Which Spread Is Better for My Heart—Butter or Margarine?" Mayo Clinic, accessed June 1, 2018, https://www.mayoclinic.org/healthy-lifestyle/ nutrition-and-healthy-eating/expert-answers/butter-vs-margarine/faq-20058152.

25. "*Trans* Fats," American Heart Association, accessed August 4, 2018, https://healthyfor good.heart.org/Eat-smart/Articles/Trans-Fat.

26. L. Pimpin, J. H. Y. Wu, H. Haskelberg, et al., "Is Butter Back? A Systematic Review and Meta-analysis of Butter Consumption and Risk of Cardiovascular Disease, Diabetes, and Total Mortality," *PLoS ONE* 11, no. 6 (June 29, 2016): e0158118, https://doi .org/10.1371/journal.pone.0158118.

27. "Artificial Sweeteners and Other Sugar Substitutes," Mayo Clinic, accessed August 4, 2018, https://www.mayoclinic.org/healthy-lifestyle/nutrition-and-healthy-eating/in -depth/art-20046936.

28. J. Suez, T. Korem, D. Zeevi, et al., "Artificial Sweeteners Induce Glucose Intolerance by Altering the Gut Microbiota," *Nature* 514 (October 9, 2014): 181–86, https://doi .org/10.1038/nature13793.

29. K. R. Tandel, "Sugar Substitutes: Health Controversy over Perceived Benefits," *Journal of Pharmacology & Pharmacotherapeutics* 2, no. 4 (2011): 236–43, https://doi .org/10.4103/0976-500X.85936.

30. M. B. Azad, A. M. Abou-Setta, B. F. Chauhan, et al., "Nonnutritive Sweeteners and Cardiometabolic Health: A Systematic Review and Meta-analysis of Randomized Controlled Trials and Prospective Cohort Studies," *CMAJ* 189, no. 28 (July 17, 2017): E929-E939, https://doi.org/10.1503/cmaj.161390.

31. "Teflon and Perfluorooctanoic Acid (PFOA)," American Cancer Society, last updated January 5, 2016, https://www.cancer.org/cancer/cancer-causes/teflon-and-perfluorooctanoic-acid-pfoa.html.

32. P. Harber, K. Saechao, and C. Boomus, "Diacetyl-Induced Lung Disease," *Toxicological Reviews* 25, no. 4 (December 2006): 261–72, https://doi.org/10.2165/00139709-200625040-00006.

33. "Public Health Aspects of the Use of Bovine Somatotrophin—15–16 March 1999," accessed August 4, 2018, https://ec.europa.eu/food/sites/food/files/safety/docs/sci-com_scv_out19_en.pdf.

34. Ibid. European Commission, "Report on Public Health Aspects of the Use of Bovine Somatotrophin." 15–16 March 1999. *Food Safety—From the Farm to the Fork.* https://ec.europa.eu/food/sites/food/files/safety/docs/sci-com_scv_out19_en.pdf.

35. M. Ellis, "US Obesity Rates on the Rise: 113 Million by 2022," *Medical News Today,* September 3, 2013, https://www.medicalnewstoday.com/articles/265556.php.

36. E. Weil, "Puberty Before Age 10: A New 'Normal'?" *New York Times*, March 30, 2012, https://www.nytimes.com/2012/04/01/magazine/puberty-before-age-10-a-new-normal.html?_r=0.

37. Y. Hawsawi, R. El-Gendy, C. Twelves, et al., "Insulin-Like Growth Factor—Oestradiol Crosstalk and Mammary Gland Tumourigenesis," *Biochimica et Biophysica Acta* 1836, no. 2 (December 2013): 345–53, https://doi.org/10.1016/j.bbcan.2013.10.005.

38. A. Savvani, C. Petraki, P. Msaouel, et al., "IGF-IEc Expression Is Associated with Advanced Clinical and Pathological Stage of Prostate Cancer," *Anticancer Research* 33, no. 6 (June 2013): 2441–45.

39. "Lactose Intolerance," Genetics Home Reference, accessed August 4, 2018, https://ghr.nlm.nih.gov/condition/lactose-intolerance.

40. A. Rubio-Tapia, I. D. Hill, C. P. Kelly, et al., "ACG Clinical Guidelines: Diagnosis and Management of Celiac Disease," *American Journal of Gastroenterology* 108, no. 5 (May 2013): 656–76, https://doi.rg/10.1038/ajg.2013.79.

41. N. Shute, "Gluten Goodbye: One-Third of Americans Say They're Trying to Shun It," National Public Radio, March 9, 2013, http://www.npr.org/sections/thesalt/2013/03/09/173840841/gluten-goodbye-one-third-of-americans-say-theyre-trying-to-shun-it.

42. B. Niland and B. D. Cash, "Health Benefits and Adverse Effects of a Gluten-Free Diet in Non–Celiac Disease Patients," *Gastroenterology & Hepatology* 14, no. 2 (February 2018): 82–91.

43. Ibid.

44. L. Chow, "It's Official: 19 European Countries Say 'No' to GMOs," EcoWatch, October 5, 2015, https://www.ecowatch.com/its-official-19-european-countries-say-no-to-gmos-1882106434.html.

45. A. Samsel and S. Seneff, "Glyphosate's Suppression of Cytochrome P450 Enzymes and Amino Acid Biosynthesis by the Gut Microbiome: Pathways to Modern Diseases," *Entropy* 15, no. 4 (2013): 1416–63.

46. A. Samsel and S. Seneff, "Glyphosate, Pathways to Modern Diseases II: Celiac Sprue and Gluten Intolerance," *Interdisciplinary Toxicology* 6, no. 4 (December 2013): 159–84, https://doi.org/10.2478/intox-2013-0026.

47. F. T. K. Basu, B. Ooraikul, "Studies on Germination Conditions and Antioxidant Contents of Wheat Grain," *International Journal of Food Sciences and Nutrition* 52, no. 4 (July 2001): 319–30.

48. K. P. Parameswaran and S. Sadasivam, "Changes in the Carbohydrates and Nitrogenous Components During Germination of Proso Millet, *Panicum miliaceum,*" *Plant Foods for Human Nutrition* 45, no. 2 (February 1994): 97–102.

49. K. Gunnars, "Why Modern Wheat Is Worse Than Older Wheat," Healthline, February 2, 2014, https://www.healthline.com/nutrition/modern-wheat-health-nightmare.

50. T. L. Greer, J. M. Trombello, C. D. Rethorst, et al., "Improvements in Psychosocial Functioning and Health-Related Quality of Life Following Exercise Augmentation in Patients with Treatment Response but Nonremitted Major Depressive Disorder: Results from the TREAD Study," *Depression and Anxiety* 33, no. 9 (September 2016): 870–81.

51. F. W. Booth, C. K. Roberts, and M. J. Laye, "Lack of Exercise Is a Major Cause of Chronic Diseases," *Comprehensive Physiology* 2, no. 2 (April 2012): 1143–1211, https://doi.org/10.1002/cphy.c110025.

52. J. H. Goedecke and L. K. Micklesfield, "The Effect of Exercise on Obesity, Body Fat Distribution and Risk for Type 2 Diabetes," *Medicine and Sport Science* 60 (2014): 82–93, https://doi.org/10.1159/000357338.

53. C. J. Lavie, R. Arena, D. L. Swift, et al., "Exercise and the Cardiovascular System: Clinical Science and Cardiovascular Outcomes," *Circulation Research* 117, no. 2 (July 3, 2015): 207–19, https://doi.org/10.1161/CIRCRESAHA.117.305205.

54. M. G. Wilson, G. M. Ellison, and N. T. Cable, "Basic Science Behind the Cardiovascular Benefits of Exercise," *Heart* 101, no. 10 (May 15, 2015): 758–65, https://doi.org/10.1136/heartjnl-2014-306596.

55. S. Y. Pan and M. DesMeules, "Energy Intake, Physical Activity, Energy Balance, and Cancer: Epidemiologic Evidence," in *Cancer Epidemiology,* M. Verma, ed., vol. 472, *Methods in Molecular Biology* (New York: Humana Press, 2009), 191–215, https://doi.org/10.1007/978-1-60327-492-0_8.

56. Ajibola I. Abioye, Majeed O. Odesanya, Asanat I. Abioye, et al., "Physical Activity and Risk of Gastric Cancer: A Meta-analysis of Observational Studies," *British Journal of Sports Medicine* 49, no. 4 (February 2015): 224–29, https://doi.org/10.1136/bjsports-2013-092778.

57. G. Behrens, C. Jochem, D. Schmid, et al., "Physical Activity and Risk of Pancreatic Cancer: A Systematic Review and Meta-analysis," *European Journal of Epidemiology* 30, no. 4 (April 2015): 279–98, https://doi.org/10.1007/s10654-015-0014-9.

58. M. I. Carter and P. S. Hinton, "Physical Activity and Bone Health," *Missouri Medicine* 111, no. 1 (January–February 2014): 59–64.

59. C. Bouchard, S. N. Blair, and P. T. Katzmarzyk, "Less Sitting, More Physical Activity, or Higher Fitness?" *Mayo Clinic Proceedings* 90, no. 11 (November 2015): 1533–40, https://doi.org/10.1016/j.mayocp.2015.08.005.

60. H. S. Friedman, "We're Not Really Living Much Longer," HuffPost, April 24, 2011, https://www.huffingtonpost.com/howard-s-friedman-phd/were-not-really-living-mu_b_852940.html.

61. M. J. Orlich, P. N. Singh, J. Sabaté, et al., "Vegetarian Dietary Patterns and Mortality in the Adventist Health Study 2," *JAMA International Medicine* 173, no. 13 (July 8, 2013): 1230–38.

Chapter 4: What You Need to Know Before You Start the Essential Oils Diet

1. M. D. Klok, S. Jakobsdottir, and M. L. Drent, "The Role of Leptin and Ghrelin in the Regulation of Food Intake and Body Weight in Humans: A Review," *Obesity Reviews* 8, no. 1 (January 2007): 21–34, https://doi.org/10.1111/j.1467-789X.2006.00270.x.

2. R. S. Ahima and D. A. Antwi, "Brain Regulation of Appetite and Satiety," *Endocrinology and Metabolism Clinics of North America* 37, no. 2 (December 2008): 811–23, https://doi.org/10.1016/j.ecl.2008.08.005.

3. A. Oswal and G. Yeo, "Leptin and the Control of Body Weight: A Review of Its Diverse Central Targets, Signaling Mechanisms, and Role in the Pathogenesis of Obesity," *Obesity* 18, no. 2 (February 2010): 221–29, https://doi.org/10.1038/oby.2009.228.

4. M. Lenoir, F. Serre, L. Cantin, et al., "Intense Sweetness Surpasses Cocaine Reward," PLOS ONE 2, no. 8 (August 1, 2007): e698, https://doi.org/10.1371/journal.pone.0000698.

5. C. Kosinski and F. R. Jornayvaz, "Effects of Ketogenic Diets on Cardiovascular Risk Factors: Evidence from Animal and Human Studies," *Nutrients* 9, no. 5 (2017): 517, https://doi.org/10.3390/nu9050517.

6. J. R. Rapin and N. Wiernsperger, "Possible Links Between Intestinal Permeability and Food Processing: A Potential Therapeutic Niche for Glutamine," *Clinics* 65, no. 6 (2010): 635–43, https://doi.org/10.1590/S1807-59322010000600012.

7. J. H. Ellenbroek, L. van Dijck, H. A. Töns, et al., "Long-Term Ketogenic Diet Causes Glucose Intolerance and Reduced β- and α-cell Mass but No Weight Loss in Mice," *American Journal of Physiology: Endocrinology and Metabolism* 306, no. 5 (March 1, 2014): E552–58.

8. N. Douris, T. Melman, J. M. Pecherer, et al., "Adaptive Changes in Amino Acid Metabolism Permit Normal Longevity in Mice Consuming a Low-Carbohydrate Ketogenic Diet," *Biochimica et Biophysica Acta* 1852, 10 pt. A (October 2015): 2056–65.

9. T. Watson, "Ancient Oat Discovery May Poke More Holes in Paleo Diet," *National Geographic*, September 11, 2015, https://www.nationalgeographic.com/people-and-culture/food/the-plate/2015/09/11/ancient-oat-discovery-may-poke-more-holes-in-paleo-diet/.

10. D. D. Weber, S. Aminazdeh-Gohari, and B. Kofler, "Ketogenic Diet in Cancer Therapy," *Aging* 10, no. 2 (February 2018): 164–65, https://doi.org/10.18632/aging.101382.

11. J. C. Callaway, "Hempseed as a Nutritional Resource: An Overview," *Euphytica* 140, no. 1–2 (January 2004): 65–72.

12. Ibid.

13. Ibid.

14. M. Mihoc, G. Pop, E. Alexa, et al., "Nutritive Quality of Romanian Hemp Varieties (*Cannabis sativa* L.) with Special Focus on Oil and Metal Contents of Seeds," *Chemistry Central Journal* 6, no. 1 (October 23, 2012): 122, https://doi.org/10.1186/1752-153x-6-122.

15. J. D. House, J. Neufeld, and G. Leson, "Evaluating the Quality of Protein from Hemp Seed (*Cannabis sativa* L.) Products Through the Use of the Protein Digestibility-Corrected Amino Acid Score Method," *Journal of Agricultural and Food Chemistry* 58, no. 22 (November 24, 2010): 11801–07, https://doil.org/10.1021/jf102636b.

16. B. J. Wells, A. G. Mainous, and C. J. Everett, "Association Between Dietary Arginine and C-reactive Protein," *Nutrition* 21, no. 2 (February 2005): 125–30.

17. Ibid.

18. R. Latif, "Health Benefits of Cocoa," *Current Opinion in Clinical Nutrition and Metabolic Care* 16, no. 6 (November 2103): 669–74, https://doi.org10.1097/MCO.0b013e328365a235.

19. Y. Gu, S. Yu, and J. D. Lambert, "Dietary Cocoa Ameliorates Obesity-Related Inflammation in High Fat–Fed Mice," *European Journal of Nutrition* 53, no. 1 (February 2014): 149–58, https://doi.org/10.1007/s00394-013-0510-1.

20. Luciana T. Toscano, Lydiane T. Toscano, Renate L. Tavares, et al., "Chia Induces Clinically Discrete Weight Loss and Improves Lipid Profile Only in Altered Previous Values," *Nutrición Hospitalaria* 31, no 3 (December 14, 2014): 1176–82, https://doi.org/10.3305/nh.2015.31.3.8242.

21. M. Mohammadi-Sartang, Z. Mazloom, H. Raeisi-Dehkordi, et al., "The Effect of Flaxseed Supplementation on Body Weight and Body Composition: A Systematic Review and Meta-analysis of 45 Randomized Placebo-Controlled Trials," *Obesity Reviews* 18, no. 9 (September 2017): 1096–1107, https://doi.org/10.1111/obr.12550.

22. M. Kristensen, M. G. Jensen, J. Aarestrup, et al., "Flaxseed Dietary Fibers Lower Cholesterol and Increase Fecal Fat Excretion, but Magnitude of Effect Depend on Food Type," *Nutrition & Metabolism* 9 (2012): 8, https://doi.org/10.1186/1743-7075-9-8.

23. Y. Rhee and A. Brunt, "Flaxseed Supplementation Improved Insulin Resistance in Obese Glucose Intolerant People: A Randomized Crossover Design," *Nutrition Journal* 10 (2011): 44, https://doi.org/10.1186/1475-2891-10-44.

24. M. M. Flynn and S. E. Rienert, "Comparing an Olive Oil–Enriched Diet to a Standard Lower-Fat Diet for Weight Loss in Breast Cancer Survivors: A Pilot Study," *Journal of Women's Health* 19, no. 6 (June 2010): 1155–61, https://doi.org/10.1089/jwh.2009.1759.

25. J. A. Menendez and R. Lupu, "Mediterranean Dietary Traditions for the Molecular Treatment of Human Cancer: Anti-oncogenic Actions of the Main Olive Oil's Monounsaturated Fatty Acid Oleic Acid (18:1n-9)," *Current Pharmaceutical Biotechnology* 7, no. 6 (December 2006): 495–502.

26. J. A. Menendez, L. Vellon, R. Colomer, et al., "Oleic Acid, the Main Monounsaturated Fatty Acid of Olive Oil, Suppresses Her-2/neu (erbB-2) Expression and Synergistically Enhances the Growth Inhibitory Effects of Trastuzumab (Herceptin) in Breast Cancer Cells with Her-2/neu Oncogene Amplification," *Annals of Oncology* 16, no. 3 (March 2005): 359–71.

27. S. Yoneyma, K. Miura, S. Sasaki, et al., "Dietary Intake of Fatty Acids and Serum C-reactive Protein in Japanese," *Journal of Epidemiology* 17, no. 3 (May 2007): 86–92.

28. K. L. Tuck and P. J. Hayball, "Major Phenolic Compounds in Olive Oil: Metabolism and Health Effects," *Journal of Nutritional Biochemistry* 13, no. 11 (November 2002): 636–44.

29. L. Schwingshack and G. Hoffmann, "Monounsaturated Fatty Acids, Olive Oil and Health Status: A Systematic Review and Meta-analysis of Cohort Studies," *Lipids in Health and Disease* 13 (October 2014):154, https:doi.org/10.1186/1476-511X-13-154.

30. S. Diano Z.-W. Liu, J. K. Jeong,, et al., "Peroxisome Proliferation–Associated Control of Reactive Oxygen Species Sets Melanocortin Tone and Feeding in Diet-Induced Obesity," *Nature Medicine* 17 (2011): 1121–27, https://doi.org/10.1038/nm.2421.

31. S. R. Goltz. W. W. Campbell, C. Chitchumroonchokchai, et al., "Meal Triacylglycerol Profile Modulates Postprandial Absorption of Carotenoids in Humans," *Molecular*

Nutrition & Food Research 56, no 6 (June 18, 2012): 866–77, https://doi.org/ 10.1002/ mnfr.201100687.

32. L. Pimpin, J. H. Y. Wu, H. Haskelberg, et al., "Is Butter Back? A Systematic Review and Meta-analysis of Butter Consumption and Risk of Cardiovascular Disease, Diabetes, and Total Mortality," *PLoS ONE* 11, no. 6 (June 29, 2016): e0158118, https://doi .org/10.1371/journal.pone.0158118.

33. L. J. James, M. P. Funnell, and S. Milner, "An Afternoon Snack of Berries Reduces Subsequent Energy Intake Compared to an Isoenergetic Confectionary Snack," *Appetite* 95 (December 1, 2015): 132–37, https://doi.org/10.1016/j.appet.2015.07.005.

34. T. Tsuda, "Recent Progress in Anti-obesity and Anti-diabetes Effect of Berries," *Antioxidants* 5, no. 2 (June 2016): 13, https://doi.org/10.3390/antiox5020013.

35. N. Z. Unlu, T. Bohn, S. K. Clinton, et al., "Carotenoid Absorption from Salad and Salsa by Humans Is Enhanced by the Addition of Avocado or Avocado Oil," *Journal of Nutrition* 135, no. 3 (March 1, 2005): 431–36, https://doi.org/10.1093/jn/135.3.431.

36. M. Wien, E. Haddad, K. Oda, et al., "A Randomized 3x3 Crossover Study to Evaluate the Effect of Hass Avocado Intake on Post-ingestive Satiety, Glucose and Insulin Levels, and Subsequent Energy Intake in Overweight Adults," *Nutrition Journal* 12 (November 27, 2013): 155.

37. Ibid.

38. C. L. Kien, J. Y. Bunn, C. L. Tompkins, et al., "Substituting Dietary Monounsaturated Fat for Saturated Fat Is Associated with Increased Daily Physical Activity and Resting Energy Expenditure and with Changes in Mood," *American Journal of Clinical Nutrition* 97, no. 4 (April 2013): 689–97, https://doi.org/10.3945/ajcn.112.051730.

39. K. Fujioka, F. Greenway, J. Sheard, et al., "The Effects of Grapefruit on Weight and Insulin Resistance: Relationship to the Metabolic Syndrome," *Journal of Medicinal Food* 9, no. 1 (Spring 2006): 49–54.

40. "Grapefruit Oil and Medication," Tisserand Institute, accessed August 5, 2018, http:// tisserandinstitute.org/learn-more/grapefruit-oil-and-medication.

41. "Feeling Great with Cruciferous Vegetables," World's Healthiest Foods (George Mateljan Foundation), accessed August 5, 2018, http://www.whfoods.com/genpage .php?tname=btnews&dbid=125.

42. *The Linus Pauling Institute Research Newsletter,* Spring/Summer 2006, accessed August 5, 2018, https://lpi.oregonstate.edu/sites/lpi.oregonstate.edu/files/pdf/newsletters/ss06 .pdf.

43. "Cruciferous Vegetables and Cancer Prevention," National Cancer Institute, reviewed June 7, 2012, https://www.cancer.gov/about-cancer/causes-prevention/risk/diet/ cruciferous-vegetables-fact-sheet.

44. J. De Noia, "Defining Powerhouse Fruits and Vegetables: A Nutrient Density Approach," Centers for Disease Control and Prevention, last updated June 5, 2014, https:// www.cdc.gov/pcd/issues/2014/13_0390.htm.

45. Y.-J. Chen, M. A. Wallig, and E. H. Jeffery, "Dietary Broccoli Lessens Development of Fatty Liver and Liver Cancer in Mice Given Diethylnitrosamine and Fed a Western or Control Diet," *Journal of Nutrition* 146, no. 3 (March 1, 2016): 542–50, https://doi .org/10.3945/jn.115.228148.

46. F. Vallejo, F. Tomas-Barberan, and C. Garcia-Viguera, "Health-Promoting Compounds in Broccoli as Influenced by Refrigerated Transport and Retail Sale Period," *Journal of Agricultural and Food Chemistry* 51, no. 10 (May 7, 2003): 3029–34.

47. C. L. Jackson and F. B. Hu, "Long-Term Associations of Nut Consumption with Body Weight and Obesity," *American Journal of Clinical Nutrition* 100, suppl. 1 (2014): 408S–11S, https://doi.org/10.3945/ajcn.113.071332.

48. E. Ros, M. A. Martínez-González, R. Estruch, et al., "Mediterranean Diet and Cardiovascular Health: Teachings of the PREDIMED Study, *Advances in Nutrition* 5, no. 3 (May 2014): 330S–36S, https://doi.org/10.3945/an.113.005389.

49. H. Jamshed, F. A. T. Sultan, R. Iqbal, et al., "Dietary Almonds Increase Serum HDL Cholesterol in Coronary Artery Disease Patients in a Randomized Controlled Trial," *Journal of Nutrition* 145, no. 19 (October 2015): 2287–92, https://doi.org/10.3945/jn.114.207944.

50. S. Y. Tan and R. D. Mattes, "Appetitive, Dietary and Health Effects of Almonds Consumed with Meals or as Snacks: A Randomized, Controlled Trial," *European Journal of Clinical Nutrition* 67 (2013): 1205–14, https://doi.org/10.1038/ejcn.2013.184.

51. J. F. Ruisinger, C. A. Gibson, J. M. Backes, et al., "Statins and Almonds to Lower Lipoproteins (the STALL Study)," *Journal of Clinical Lipidology* 9 no. 1 (January–February 2015): 58–64, https://doi.org/10.1016/j.jacl.2014.10.001.

52. Tan and Mattes, "Appetitive, Dietary and Health Effects of Almonds Consumed with Meals or as Snacks: A Randomized, Controlled Trial."

53. C. E. Berryman, S. G. West, J. A. Fleming, et al., "Effects of Daily Almond Consumption on Cardiometabolic Risk and Abdominal Adiposity in Healthy Adults with elevated LDL-Cholesterol: A Randomized Controlled Trial," *Journal of the American Heart Association* 4, no. 1 (January 5, 2015): e000993, https://doi.org/10.1161/JAHA.114.000993.

54. M. A. Wein, J. M. Sabaté, D. N. Iklé, et al., "Almonds vs Complex Carbohydrates in a Weight Reduction Program," *International Journal of Obesity Related Metabolic Disorders* 27, no. 11 (November 2003): 1365–72.

55. "Food and Nutrition Information Center," USDA National Agricultural Library, accessed August 5, 2018, http://www.nal.usda.gov/fnic.

56. S. Torabian, E. Haddad, S. Rajaram, et al., "Acute Effect of Nut Consumption on Plasma Total Polyphenols, Antioxidant Capacity and Lipid Peroxidation," *Journal of Human Nutrition and Dietetics* 22, no. 1 (February 2009): 64–71, https://doi.org/10.1111/j.1365-277X.2008.00923.x.

57. E. J. Reverri, J. M. Randolph, F. M. Steinberg, et al., "Black Beans, Fiber, and Antioxidant Capacity Pilot Study: Examination of Whole Foods *vs.* Functional Components on Postprandial Metabolic, Oxidative Stress, and Inflammation in Adults with Metabolic Syndrome," *Nutrients* 7, no. 8 (2015): 6139–54, https://doi.org/10.3390/nu7085273.

58. M. Migliozzi, D. Thavarajah, P. Thavarajah, et al., "Lentil and Kale: Complementary Nutrient-Rich Whole Food Sources to Combat Micronutrient and Calorie Malnutrition," *Nutrients* 7, no. 11 (2015): 9285–98, https://doi.org/10.3390/nu7115471.

59. Ibid.

60. Ibid.

61. "Omega-3 Content of Frequently Consumed Seafood Products," Seafood Health Facts: Making Smart Choices, accessed August 5, 2018, https://www.seafoodhealthfacts.org/seafood-nutrition/healthcare-professionals/omega-3-content-frequently-consumed-seafood-products.

62. "Omega-3 Fatty Acids," National Institutes for Health, last updated June 6, 2018, https://ods.od.nih.gov/factsheets/Omega3FattyAcids-HealthProfessionals.

63. A. Ramel, J. A. Martinez, M. Kiely, et al., "Effects of Weight Loss and Seafood Consumption on Inflammation Parameters in Young, Overweight and obese European men and women during 8 weeks of Energy Restriction," *European Journal of Clinical Nutrition* 64, no. 9 (September 2010): 987–93, https://doi.org/10.1038/ejcn.2010.99.

64. "Tea and Cancer Prevention," NIH National Cancer Institute, accessed August 5, 2018, http://www.cancer.gov/cancertopics/factsheet/prevention/tea.

65. T. Nagago, Y. Komine, S. Sogga, et al., "Ingestion of a Tea Rich in Catechins Leads to a Reduction in Body Fat and Malondialdehyde-Modified LDL in Men," *American Journal of Clinical Nutrition* 81, no. 1 (January 2005): 122–29.

66. D. J. Weiss and C. R. Anderton, "Determination of Catechins in Matcha Green Tea by Micellar Electrokinetic Chromatography," *Journal of Chromatography* 1011, no. 1–2 (September 5, 2003): 173–80.

67. T. Ichinose, S. Nomura, Y. Someya, et al., "The Effect of Endurance Training Supplemented with Green Tea Extract on Substrate Metabolism During Exercise in Humans," *Scandinavian Journal of Medicine and Science in Sports* 21, no. 4 (August 2011): 598–605.

68. I. S. Hong, H. Y. Lee, and H. P. Kim, "Anti-oxidative Effects of Rooibos Tea *(Aspalathus linearis)* on Immobilization-Induced Oxidative Stress in Rat Brain," *PLoS ONE* 9, no. 1 (January 21, 2014): e87061, https://doi.org/10.1371/journal.pone.0087061.

Chapter 5: The 30-Day Essential Fast Track: Form New Habits and Kick-start Wieght Loss

1. "Pork Chops and Ground Pork Contaminated with Bacteria," *Consumer Reports,* January 2013, accessed August 6, 2018, https://www.consumerreports.org/cro/magazine/2013/01/what-s-in-that-pork/index.htm.

2. A. A. Baer, M. J. Miller, A. C. Dilger, "Pathogens of Interest to the Pork Industry: A Review of Research on Interventions to Assure Food Safety," *Comprehensive Reviews in Food Science and Food Safety* 12, no. 2 (March 2013): 183–217, https://doi.org/10.1111/1541-4337.12001.

3. M. Mataragas, P. N. Skandamis, and E. H. Drosinos, "Risk Profiles of Pork and Poultry Meat and Risk Ratings of Various Pathogen/Product Combinations," *International Journal of Food Microbi8ology* 126, no. 1–2 (August 15, 2008): 1–12, https://doi.org/10.1016/j.ijfoodmicro.2008.05.014.

4. A. A. Baer, M. J. Miller, and A. C. Dilger, "Pathogens of Interest to the Pork Industry: A Review of Research on Interventions to Assure Food Safety," *Comprehensive Reviews in Food Science and Food Safety* 12, no. 2 (March 2013): 183–217, https://doi.org/10.1111/1541-4337.12001.

5. F. Gagnon, T. Tremblay, J. Rouette, et al., "Chemical Risks Associated with Consumption of Shellfish Harvested on the North Shore of the St. Lawrence River's Lower Estuary," *Environmental Health Perspectives* 112, no. 8 (June 2004): 883–88.

6. E. M. Matheson, A. G. Mainous III, E. G. Hill, et al., "Shellfish Consumption and Risk of Coronary Heart Disease," *Journal of the American Dietetic Association* 109, no. 8 (August 2009): 1422–26, https://doi.org/10.1016/j.jada.2009.05.007.

7. G. Traversy and J.-P. Chaput, "Alcohol Consumption and Obesity: An Update," *Current Obesity Reports* 4, no. 1 (March 2015): 122–30, https://doi.org/10.1007/s13679-014-0129-4.

8. "Xylitol," WebMD, accessed August 6, 2018, http://www.webmd.com/vitamins-supplements/ingredientmono-996-xylitol.aspx?activeingredientid=996&activeingredientname=xylitol.

9. I. Rustenbeck, V. Lier-Glaubitz, M. Willenborg, et al., "Effect of Chronic Coffee Consumption on Weight Gain and Glycaemia in a Mouse Model of Obesity and Type 2 Diabetes," *Nutrition & Diabetes* 4, no. 6 (June 2014): e123, https://doi.org/10.1038/nutd.2014.19.

10. S. Bidel, G. Hu, J. Sundvall, et al., "Effects of Coffee Consumption on Glucose Tolerance, Serum Glucose and Insulin Levels—A Cross-Sectional Analysis," *Hormone and Metabolic Research* 38, no. 1 (January 2006): 38–43, https://doi.org/10.1055/s-2006-924982.

11. K. R. Sajadi-Ernazarova and R. J. Hamilton, "Caffeine Withdrawal," National Center for Biotechnology Information, last updated May 11, 2017, https://www.ncbi.nlm.nih.gov/books/NBK430790.

12. S. E. Meredith, L. M. Juliano, J. R. Hughes, et al., "Caffeine Use Disorder: A Comprehensive Review and Research Agenda," *Journal of Caffeine Research* 3, no. 3 (September 2013): 114–30, https://doi.org/10.1089/jcr.2013.0016.

13. C. Drake, T. Roehrs, J. Shambroom, et al., "Caffeine Effects on Sleep Taken 0, 3, or 6 Hours Before Going to Bed," *Journal of Clinical Sleep Medicine* 9, no. 11 (November 15, 2013): 1195–1200, https://doi.org/10.5664/jcsm.3170.

14. K. Ishiguro, R. Kurata, Y. Shimada, et al., "Effects of a Sweet Potato Protein Digest on Lipid Metabolism in Mice Administered a High-Fat Diet," *Heliyon* 2, no. 12 (December 7, 2017), https://doi.org/10.1016/j.heliyon.2016.e00201.

15. Z. Radak, Z. Zhao, E. Koltai, et al., "Oxygen Consumption and Usage During Physical Exercise: The Balance Between Oxidative Stress and ROS-Dependent Adaptive Signaling," *Antioxidants & Redox Signaling* 18, no. 10 (April 1, 2013): 1208–46, https://doi.org/10.1089/ars.2011.4498.

16. C. Álvarez, R. Ramírez-Campillo, R. Ramírez-Vélez, et al., "Metabolic Effects of Resistance or High-Intensity Interval Training Among Glycemic Control-Nonresponsive Children with Insulin Resistance," *International Journal of Obesity* 42, no. 1 (January 2018): 79–87, https://doi.org/10.1038/ijo.2017.177.

17. C. Álvarez, R. Ramírez-Campillo, R. Ramírez-Vélez, et al., "Prevalence of Nonresponders for Glucose Control Markers After 10 Weeks of High-Intensity Interval Training in Adult Women with Higher and Lower Insulin Resistance," *Frontiers in Physiology* 8 (2017): 479, https://doi.org/10.3389/fphys.2017.00479.

18. T. E. Keshel and R.H. Coker, "Exercise Training and Insulin Resistance: A Current Review," *Journal of Obesity and Weight Loss Therapy* (July 2015): S5-003, https://doi.org/10.4172/2165-7904.S5-003.

19. "Metabolism and Weight Loss: How You Burn Calories," Mayo Clinic, accessed August 6, 2018, https://www.mayoclinic.org/healthy-lifestyle/weight-loss/in-depth/metabolism/art-20046508.

20. E. A. Marques, J. Mota, and J. Carvalho, "Exercise Effects on Bone Mineral Density in Older Adults: A Meta-analysis of Randomized Controlled Trials," *Age* 34, no. 6 (December 2012): 1493–1515, https://doi.org/10.1007/s11357-011-9311-8.

21. D. Solanki and A. M. Lane, "Relationships Between Exercise as a Mood Regulation Strategy and Trait Emotional Intelligence," *Asian Journal of Sports Medicine* 1, no. 4 (2010): 195–200.

22. K. M. Diaz, V. J. Howard, B. Hutto, et al., "Patterns of Sedentary Behavior and Mortality in U.S. Middle-Aged and Older Adults: A National Cohort Study," *Annals of Internal Medicine* 167, no. 7 (2017): 465–75, https://doi.org/10.7326/M17-0212.

23. "Sedentary Time May Raise Heart Disease Risk—Sit Less, Move More," American

Heart Association, August 15, 2017, http://newsroom.heart.org/news/sedentary-time-may-raise-heart-disease-risk-sit-less-move-more.

24. B. M. Popkin, K. E. D'Anci, and I. H. Rosenberg, "Water, Hydration, and Health," *Nutrition Reviews* 68, no. 8 (August 1, 2010: 439–58, https://doi.org/10.1111/j.1753-4887.2010.00304.x.

25. R. Muckelbauer, G. Sarganas, A. Grüneis, et al., "Association Between Water Consumption and Body Weight Outcomes: A Systematic Review," *American Journal of Clinical Nutrition* 98, no. 2 (August 1, 2013): 282–99, https://doi.org/10.3945/ajcn.112.055061.

26. M. Boschmann, J. Steiniger, U. Hille, et al., "Water-Induced Thermogenesis," *Journal of Clinical Endocrinology and Metabolism* 88, no .12 (December 2003): 6015–19, https:doi.org/10.1210/jc.2003-030780.

27. "Skin Turgor," MedlinePlus, accessed August 6, 2018, https://medlineplus.gov/ency/article/003281.htm.

28. K. Nagai, A. Niijima, Y. Horii, et al., "Olfactory Stimulatory with Grapefruit and Lavender Oils Change Autonomic Nerve Activity and Physiological Function," *Autonomic Neuroscience: Basic and Clinical* 185 (October 2014): 29–35, https://doi.org/10.1016/j.autneu.2014.06.005.

29. K.-H. Kim, Y. H. Kim, J. E. Son, et al., "Intermittent Fasting Promotes Adipose Thermogenesis and Metabolic Homeostasis via VEGF-mediated Alternative Activation of Macrophage," *Cell Research* 27, no. 11 (2017): 1309–26, https://doi.org/10.1038/cr.2017.126.

30. M. C. Klempel, C. M. Kroeger, S. Bhutani, et al., "Intermittent Fasting Combined with Calorie Restriction Is Effective for Weight Loss and Cardio-protection in Obese Women," *Nutrition Journal* 11 (November 21, 2012): 98, https://doi.org/10.1186/1475-2891-11-98.

31. A. D. Welling, "Colon Cleansing and Body Detoxification: Any Evidence of Benefit or Harm?" *American Family Physician* 81, no. 3 (February 1, 2010): 337, accessed August 6, 2018, https://www.aafp.org/afp/2010/0201/p337.html.

32. B. M. Altevogt and H. R. Colten, eds., *Sleep Disorders and Sleep Deprivation: An Unmet Public Health Problem* (Washington, DC: National Academies Press, 2006).

33. D. Yin, "Is Carbonyl Detoxification an Important Anti-aging Process During Sleep?" *Medical Hypotheses* 54, no. 4 (April 2000): 519–22, https://doi.org/10.1054/mehy.1999.0889.

34. J. E. Carroll, T. E. Seeman, R. Olmstead, et al., "Improved Sleep Quality in Older Adults with Insomnia Reduces Biomarkers of Disease Risk: Pilot Results from a Randomized Controlled Comparative Efficacy Trial," *Psychoneuroendocrinology* 55 (May 2015): 184–92, https://doi.org/10.1016/j.psyneuen.2015.02.010.

35. S. R. Patel and F. B. Hu, "Short Sleep Duration and Weight Gain: A Systematic Review," *Obesity* 16, no. 3 (March 2008): 643–53.

36. S. R. Patel, A. Malhotra, D. P. White, et al., "Association Between Reduced Sleep and Weight Gain in Women," *American Journal of Epidemiology* 164, no. 10 (November 15, 2006): 947–54.

37. M. O. Melancon, D. Lorrain, and I. J. Dionne, "Exercise and Sleep in Aging: Emphasis on Serotonin," *Pathologie-Biologie* 62, no. 5 (October 2014): 276–83, https:doi.org/10.1016/j.patbio.2014.07.004.

38. P. H. Koulivand, M. K. Ghadiri, and A. Gorji, "Lavender and the Nervous System," *Evidence-Based Complementary and Alternative Medicine* 2013 (2013), https:doi.org/10.1155/2013/681304.

39. H. Woelk and S. Schläfke, "A Multi-center, Double-Blind, Randomized Study of the Lavender Oil Preparation Silexan in Comparison to Lorazepam for Generalized Anxiety Disorder," *Phytomedicine* 17, no. 2 (February 2010): 94–99, https://doi.org/10.1016/j.phymed.2009.10.006.

40. B. J. Malcolm and K. Tallian, "Essential Oil of Lavender in Anxiety Disorders: Ready for Prime Time?" *Mental Health Clinician* 7, no. 4 (July 2017): 147–55, https://doi.org/10.9740/mhc.2017.07.147.

41. Koulivand, Ghadiri, and Gorji, "Lavender and the Nervous System."

42. E. S. LeBlanc, J. H. Rizo, K. L. Pedula, et al., "Associations Between 25-Hydroxyvitamin D and Weight Gain in Elderly Women," *Journal of Women's Health* 21, no. 10 (October 2012): 1066–73, https://doi.org/10.1089/jwh.2012.3506.

43. Z.-T.-N. H. Mehmood and D. Papandreou, "An Updated Mini Review of Vitamin D and Obesity: Adipogenesis and Inflammation State," *Open Access Macedonian Journal of Medical Sciences* 4, no. 3 (2016): 526–32, https://doi.org/10.3889/oamjms.2016.103.

44. K. J. Reid et al., "Timing and Intensity of Light Correlate with Body Weight in Adults," *PLoS ONE* 9, no. 4 (2014): e92251, https://doi.org/10.1371/journal.pone.0092251.

45. A. J. van Ballegooijen, S. Pilz, A. Tomaschitz, et al., "The Synergistic Interplay Between Vitamins D and K for Bone and Cardiovascular Health: A Narrative Review," *International Journal of Endocrinology* 2017 (2017): 7454376, https://doi.org/10.1155/2017/7454376.

Chapter 6: Essential Oils for Weight-Loss Support

1. J. B. Mowry, D. A. Spyker, L. R. Cantilena Jr., et al., "2013 Annual Report of the American Association of Poison Control Centers' National Poison Data System (NPDS): 31st Annual Report," *Clinical Toxicology* 52, no. 10 (December 2014): 1032–283, https://doi.org/10.3109/15563650.2.

2. M. Nasri, S. Fayazi, S. Jahani, et al., "The Effect of Topical Olive Oil on the Healing of Foot Ulcer in Patients with Type 2 Diabetes: A Double-Blind Randomized Clinical Trial Study in Iran," *Journal of Diabetes & Metabolic Disorders* 14 (2015): 38, https://doi.org/10.1186/s40200-015-0167-9.

3. K. G. Nevin and T. Rajamohan, "Effect of Topical Application of Virgin Coconut Oil on Skin Components and Antioxidant Status During Dermal Wound Healing in Young Rats," *Skin Pharmacology and Physiology* 23, no. 6 (2010): 290–97, https://doi.org/10.1159/000313516.

4. Z. Ahmed, "The Uses and Properties of Almond Oil," *Complementary Therapies in Clinical Practice* 16, no. 1 (February 2010): 10–12, https:doi.org/10.1016/j.ctcp.2009.06.015.

5. R. R. Habashy, A. B. Abdel-Naim, A. E. Khalifa, et al., "Anti-inflammatory Effects of Jojoba Liquid Wax in Experimental Models," *Pharmacological Research* 51, no. 2 (February 2005): 95–105.

6. A. Gupta, P. S. Sharma, B. M. K. S. Tilakratne, et al., "Studies on Physico-chemical Characteristics and Fatty Acid Composition of Wild Apricot *(Prunus armeniaca)* Kernel Oil," *Indian Journal of Natural Products and Resources* 3, no. 3 (September 2012): 366–70.

7. B. S. Nayak, S. S. Raju, A. V. Chalapathi Rao, "Wound Healing Activity of *Persea americana* (Avocado) Fruit: A Preclinical Study on Rats," *Journal of Wound Care* 17, no. 3 (March 2008): 123–26.

8. H. Lutterodt, M. Slavin, M. Whent, et al., "Fatty Acid Composition, Oxidative Stability, Antioxidant and Antiproliferative Properties of Selected Cold-Pressed Grape

Seed Oils and Flours," *Food Chemistry* 128, no. 2 (September 2011): 391–99, https://doi .org/10.1016/j.foodchem.2011.03.040.

9. R. H. Foster, G. Hardy, and R. G. Alany, "Borage Oil in the Treatment of Atopic Dermatitis," *Nutrition* 26, no. 7–8 (July–August 2010): 708–18, https://doi.org/10.1016/j .nut.2009.10.014.

10. F. Farzaneh, S. Fatehi, and R.-M. Sohrabi, "The Effect of Oral Evening Primrose Oil on Menopausal Hot Flashes: A Randomized Clinical Trial," *Archives of Gynecology and Obstetrics* 288, no. 5 (November 2013): 1075–79, https://doi.org/10.1007/ s00404-013-2852-6.

11. J. Shen, A. Niijima, M. Tanida, et al., "Olfactory Stimulation with Scent of Grapefruit Oil Affects Autonomic Nerves, Lipolysis and Appetite in Rats," *Neuroscience Letters* 380, no. 3 (June 2005): 289–94.

12. R. Meerman and A. J. Brown, "When Somebody Loses Weight, Where Does the Fat Go?" *BMJ* 349, no. 7988 (December 2014): 37–38, https://doi.org/10.1136/bmj.g7257.

13. Nagai, Niijima, Horii, et al., "Olfactory Stimulatory with Grapefruit and Lavender Oils" (see chap. 5, n. 28).

14. Shen, Niijima, Tanida, et al., "Olfactory Stimulation with Scent of Grapefruit Oil."

15. H. J. Kim, "Effect of Aromatherapy Massage on Abdominal Fat And Body Image for Post-menopausal Women," *Taehan Kanho Hakhoe Chi* 37, no. 4 (2007): 603–12.

16. S. Asnaashari, A. Delazar, B. Habibi, et al., "Essential Oil from *Citrus aurantifolia* Prevents Ketotifen-Induced Weight-Gain in Mice," *Phytotherapy Research* 24, no. 12 (November 2010): 1893–97, https://doi.org/10.1002/ptr.3227.

17. B. Mizrahi, L. Shapira, A. Domb, et al., "Citrus Oil and MgCl2 as Antibacterial and Anti-inflammatory Agents," *Journal of Periodontology* 77, no. 6 (2006): 963– 68, https:// doi.org/10.1902/jop.2006.050278.

18. W.-J. Yoon, N. H. Lee, and C.-G. Jyun, "Limonene Suppresses Lipopolysaccharide-Induced Production of Nitric Oxide, Prostaglandin E2, and Pro-inflammatory Cytokines in RAW 264.7 Macrophages," *Journal of Oleo Science* 59, no. 8 (2010): 415–21, https://doi.org/10.5650/jos.59.415.

19. E. E. Revay, A. Junnila, R.-D. Xue, et al., "Evaluation of Commercial Products for Personal Protection Against Mosquitoes," *Acta Tropica* 125, no. 2 (February 2013): 226–30, https://doi.org/10.1016/j.actatropica.2012.10.009.

20. E. Schmidt, S. Bail, G. Buchbauer, et al., "Chemical Composition, Olfactory Evaluation and Antioxidant Effects of Essential Oil from *Mentha × piperita*," *Natural Product Communications* 4, no. 8 (August 2009): 1107–12.

21. J. A. Reed, J. Almeida, B. Wershing, et al., "Effects of Peppermint Scent on Appetite Control and Caloric Intake," *Appetite* 51, no. 2 (September 2008): 393, https://doi .org/10.1016/j.appet.2008.04.196.

22. G. K. Jayaprakasha and L. J. M. Rao, "Chemistry, Biogenesis, and Biological Activities of *Cinnamomum zeylanicum*," *Critical Reviews in Food Science and Nutrition* 51, no. 6 (July 2011): 547–62, https://doi.org/10.1080/10408391003699550.

23. P. A. Davis and W. Yokoyama, "Cinnamon Intake Lowers Fasting Blood Glucose: Meta-analysis," *Journal of Medicinal Food* 14, no. 9 (September 2011): 884–89, https://doi .org/10.1089/jmf.2010.0180.

24. P. Subash Babu, S. Prabuseenivasan, S. Ignacimuthu, "Cinnamaldehyde—A Potential Antidiabetic Agent," *Phytomedicine* 14, no. 1 (January 2007): 15–22.

25. R. M. Hafizur, A. Hameed, M. Shukrana, et al., "Cinnamic Acid Exerts Anti-diabetic Activity by Improving Glucose Tolerance *in vivo* and by Stimulating Insulin Secretion *in vitro*," *Phytomedicine* 22, no. 2 (February 15, 2015): 297–300, https://doi.org/10.1016/j.phymed.2015.01.003.

26. N. Talpur, B. Echard, C. Ingram, et al., "Effects of a Novel Formulation of Essential Oils on Glucose-Insulin Metabolism in Diabetic and Hypertensive Rats: A Pilot Study," *Diabetes, Obesity & Metabolism* 7, no. 2 (March 2005): 193–99.

27. Ibid.

28. M. Igarashi, H. Ikei, C. Song, et al., "Effects of Olfactory Stimulation with Rose and Orange Oil on Prefrontal Cortex Activity," *Complementary Therapies in Medicine* 22, no. 6 (December 2014): 1027–31, https:doi.org/10.1016/j.ctim.2014.09.003.

29. D. Lo Furno, A. C. E. Graziano, R. Avola, et al., "A *Citrus bergamia* Extract Decreases Adipogenesis and Increases Lipolysis by Modulating PPAR Levels in Mesenchymal Stem Cells from Human Adipose Tissue," *PPAR Research* 2016, no. 4563815 (2016), https://doi.org/10.1155/2016/4563815.

30. E. Watanabe, K. Kutcha, M. Kimura, et al., "Effects of Bergamot (*Citrus bergamia* (Risso) Wright & Arn.) Essential Oil Aromatherapy on Mood States, Parasympathetic Nervous System Activity, and Salivary Cortisol Levels in 41 Healthy Females," *Forschende Komplementarmedizin* 22 (2015): 43– 49, https://doi.org/10.1159/000380989.

31. K. Fisher and C. A. Phillips, "The Effect of Lemon, Orange and Bergamot Essential Oils and Their Components on the Survival of *Campylobacter jejuni, Escherichia coli* O157, *Listeria monocytogenes, Bacillus cereus* and *Staphylococcus aureus in vitro* and in Food Systems," *Journal of Applied Microbiology* 101 (2006): 1232–40, https://doi.org/10.1111/j.1365-2672.2006.03035.x.

32. Koulivand, Ghadiri, and Gorji, "Lavender and the Nervous System."

33. J. Buckle, *Clinical Aromatherapy,* 3rd ed. (London: Churchill Livingstone, 2014), 295.

34. A. Meamarbashi and A. Rajabi, "The Effects of Peppermint on Exercise Performance," *Journal of the International Society of Sports Nutrition* 10 (2013): 15, https://doi.org/10.1186/1550-2783-10-15.

35. A. Meamarbashi, "Instant Effects of Peppermint Essential Oil on the Physiological Parameters and Exercise Performance," *Avicenna Journal of Phytomedicine* 4, no. 1 (2014): 72–78.

36. M.-C. Ou, Y.-F. Lee, C.-C. Li, et al., "The Effectiveness of Essential Oils for Patients with Neck Pain: A Randomized Controlled Study," *Journal of Alternative Complementary and Medicine* 20, no. 10 (2014): 771–79, https://doi.org/10.1089/acm.2013.0453.

37. B. Ali, N. A. Al-Wabel, S. Shams, et al., "Essential Oils Used in Aromatherapy: A Systemic Review," *Asian Pacific Journal of Tropical Biomedicine* 5, no. 8 (2015): 601–11, https://doi.org/10.1016/j.apjtb.2015.05.007.

38. N. Talpur, B. Echard, C. Ingram, et al., "Effects of a Novel Formulation of Essential Oils on Glucose-Insulin Metabolism in Diabetic and Hypertensive Rats: A Pilot Study," *Diabetes, Obesity & Metabolism* 7, no. 2 (March 2005): 193–99.

39. G. Oboh, I. A. Akinbola, A. O. Ademosun, et al., "Essential Oil from Clove Bud (*Eugenia aromatica* Kuntze) Inhibit Key Enzymes Relevant to the Management of Type-2 Diabetes and Some Pro-oxidant Induced Lipid Peroxidation in Rats Pancreas *in Vitro*," *Journal of Oleo Science* 64, no. 7 (2015): 775–82, https://doi.org/10.5650/jos.ess14274.

40. M. J. Chung, S.-Y. Cho, M. J. H. Bhuiyan, et al., "Anti-diabetic Effects of Lemon Balm (*Melissa officinalis*) Essential Oil on Glucose- and Lipid-Regulating Enzymes in Type 2

Diabetic Mice," *British Journal of Nutrition* 104, no. 2 (July 2010): 180–88, https://doi .org/10.1017/S0007114510001765.

41. G. Oboh, A. O. Ademosun, O. V. Odubanjo, et al., "Antioxidative Properties and Inhibition of Key Enzymes Relevant to Type-2 Diabetes and Hypertension by Essential Oils from Black Pepper," *Advances in Pharmacological Sciences* 2013, article ID 926047 (2013), https://doi.org/10.1155/2013/926047.

42. H.-F. Yen, C.-T. Hsieh, T.-J. Hsieh, et al., "*In vitro* Anti-diabetic Effect and Chemical Component Analysis of 29 Essential Oils Products," *Journal of Food and Drug Analysis* 23, no. 1 (March 2015): 124–29.

43. C.-H. Ni et al., "The Anxiolytic Effect of Aromatherapy on Patients Awaiting Ambulatory Surgery: A Randomized Controlled Trial," *Evidence-Based Complementary and Alternative Medicine* 2013, article ID 927419 (2013), https://doi.org/10.1155/2013/927419.

44. B. Ali, N. A. Al-Wabel, S. Shams, et al., "Essential Oils Used in Aromatherapy: A Systemic Review," *Asian Pacific Journal of Tropical Biomedicine* 5, no. 8 (2015): 601–11, https://doi.org/10.1016/j.apjtb.2015.05.007.

45. T. Hongratanaworakit and G. Buchbauer, "Relaxing Effect of Ylang Ylang Oil on Humans After Transdermal Absorption," *Phytotherapy Research* 20, no. 9 (September 2006): 758–63, https://doi.org/10.1002/ptr.1950.

46. W. N. Setzer, "Essential Oils and Anxiolytic Aromatherapy," *Natural Product Communications* 4, no. 9 (September 2009): 1305–16.

47. J. Buckle, *Clinical Aromatherapy,* 3rd ed. (London: Churchill Livingstone, 2014).

48. Ibid.

49. B. Adam, T. Liebregts, J. Best, et al., "A Combination of Peppermint Oil and Caraway Oil Attenuates the Post-inflammatory Visceral Hyperalgesia in a Rat Model," *Scandinavian Journal of Gastroenterology* 41, no. 2 (2006): 155–60, https://doi.org/10.1080 /00365520500206442.

50. Y. A. Taher, A. M. Samud, F. E. El-Taher, et al., "Experimental Evaluation of Antiinflammatory, Antinociceptive and Antipyretic Activities of Clove Oil in Mice," *Libyan Journal of Medicine*, 10 (2015), https://doi.org/10.3402/ljm.v10.28685.

51. J. Silva, W. Abebe, S. M. Sousa, et al., "Analgesic and Anti-inflammatory Effects of Essential Oils of Eucalyptus," *Journal of Ethnopharmacology* 89, no. 2–3 (2003): 277–83, https://doi.org/10.1016/j.jep.2003.09.007.

52. K. Jeena, V. B. Liju, and R. Kuttan, "Antioxidant, Anti-inflammatory and Antinociceptive Activities of Essential Oil from Ginger," *Indian Journal of Physiology and Pharmacology*, 57, no. 1 (2013): 51–62.

53. G. L. da Silva, C. Luft, A. Lunardelli, et al., "Antioxidant, Analgesic and Anti-inflammatory Effects of Lavender Essential Oil," *Anais da Academia Brasileira de Xiências*, 87, suppl. 2, (2015): 1397–408, https://doi.org/10.1590/0001-3765201520150056.

54. M.-C. Ou, Y.-F. Lee, C.-C. Li, et al., "The Effectiveness of Essential Oils for Patients with Neck Pain: A Randomized Controlled Study," *Journal of Alternative and Complementary Medicine* 20, no. 10 (2014): 771–79, https://doi.org/10.1089/acm.2013.0453.

55. A. Bukovská, Š. Cikoš, Š. Juhás, et al., "Effects of a Combination of Thyme and Oregano Essential Oils on TNBS-Induced Colitis in Mice," *Mediators of Inflammation* 2007, article ID 23296 (2007), https://doi.org/10.1155/2007/23296.

56. Z. Sun, H. Wang, J. Wang, et al., "Chemical Composition and Anti-Inflammatory, Cytotoxic and Antioxidant Activities of Essential Oil from Leaves of *Mentha piperita*

Grown in China," *PLoS ONE* 9, no. 12 (2014): e114767, https://doi.org/10.1371/journal .pone.0114767.

57. J. K. Srivastava, E. Shankar, and S. Gupta, "Chamomile: A Herbal Medicine of the Past with Bright Future," *Molecular Medicine Reports* 3, no. 6 (2010): 895–901, https://doi .org/10.3892/mmr.2010.377.

58. K. J. Koh, A. L. Pearce, G. Marshman, et al., "Tea Tree Oil Reduces Histamine-Induced Skin Inflammation," *British Journal of Dermatology* 147, no. 6 (December 2002): 1212–17, https://doi.org/10.1046/j.1365-2133.2002.05034.x.

59. Bukovská, Cikoš, Juhás, et al., "Effects of a Combination of Thyme and Oregano Essential Oils."

60. V. B. Liju, K. Jeena, R. Kuttan, "An Evaluation of Antioxidant, Anti-inflammatory, and Antinociceptive Activities of Essential Oil from *Curcuma longa* L.," *Indian Journal of Pharmacology* 43, no. 5 (2011): 526–31, https://doi.org/10.4103/0253-7613.84961.

61. J. H. Liu, G. H. Chen, H. Z. Yeh, et al., "Enteric-Coated Peppermint-Oil Capsules in the Treatment of Irritable Bowel Syndrome: A Prospective, Randomized Trial," *Journal of Gastroenterology* 32, no. 6 (December 1997): 765–68.

62. A. Thompson, D. Meah, N. Ahmed, et al., "Comparison of the Antibacterial Activity of Essential Oils and Extracts of Medicinal and Culinary Herbs to Investigate Potential New Treatments for Irritable Bowel Syndrome," *BMC Complementary and Alternative Medicine* 13 (November 28, 2013): 338, https://doi.org/10.1186/1472-6882-13-338.

63. D. Thapa, P. Louis, R. Losa, et al., "Essential Oils Have Different Effects on Human Pathogenic and Commensal Bacteria in Mixed Faecal Fermentations Compared with Pure Cultures," *Microbiology* 161, pt. 2 (February 2015): 441–49, https://doi.org/10.1099/ mic.0.000009.

64. S. Agah, A. M. Taleb, R. Moeini, et al., "Cumin Extract for Symptom Control in Patients with Irritable Bowel Syndrome: A Case Series," *Middle East Journal of Digestive Diseases* 5, no. 4 (2013): 217–22.

Chapter 7: Forever Transform Your Life and Health with the Essential Lifestyle

1. A. J. van Ballegooijen, S. Pilz, A. Tomaschitz, et al., "The Synergistic Interplay Between Vitamins D and K for Bone and Cardiovascular Health: A Narrative Review," *International Journal of Endocrinology* 2017 (2017): 7454376, https://doi.org/10.1155/2017 /7454376.

2. M. J. J. Ronis, K. Mercer, and J.-R. Chen, "Effects of Nutrition and Alcohol Consumption on Bone Loss," *Current Osteoporosis Reports* 9, no. 2 (June 2011): 53–59, https://doi .org/10.1007/s11914-011-0049-0.

3. J. Connor, "Alcohol Consumption as a Cause of Cancer," *Addiction* 112, no. 2 (February 2017): 22228, https://doi.org/10.1111/add.13477.

4. D.-H. Lee, I.-K. Lee, K. Song, et al., "A Strong Dose-Response Relation Between Serum Concentrations of Persistent Organic Pollutants and Diabetes: Results from the National Health and Examination Survey 1999–2002," *Diabetes Care* 29, no. 7 (July 2006): 1638–44, https://doi.org/10.2337/dc06-0543.

5. E. L. Dirinck, A. C. Dirtu, M. Govindan, et al., "Exposure to Persistent Organic Pollutants: Relationship with Abnormal Glucose Metabolism and Visceral Adiposity," *Diabetes Care* 37, no. 7 (July 2014): 1951–58, https://doi.org/10.2337/dc13-2329.

6. Locke Hughes, "9 Ways Digestive Issues Can Cause Weight Gain," *Redbook,* January 18,

2018, https://www.msn.com/en-us/health/medical/9-ways-digestive-issues-can-cause
-weight-gain/ar-AAuRgvD.

7. A. P. Liou and P. J. Turnbaugh, "Antibiotic Exposure Promotes Fat Gain," *Cell Metabolism* 16, no. 4 (October 3, 2012): 408–10, https://doi.org/10.1016/j.cmet.2012.09.009.

8. O. Turta and S. Rautava, "Antibiotics, Obesity and the Link to Microbes—What Are We Doing to Our Children?" *BMC Medicine* 14 (2016): 57, https://doi.org/10.1186/s12916-016-0605-7.

9. E. T. Rogawski, J. A. Platts-Mills, J.C. Seidman, et al., "Early Antibiotic Exposure in Low-Resource Settings Is Associated with Increased Weight in the First Two Years of Life," *Journal of Pediatric Gastroenterology and Nutrition* 65, no. 3 (September 2017): 350–56, https://doi.org/10.1097/MPG.0000000000001640.

10. R. Ramallal, E. Toledo, J. A. Martínez, et al., "Inflammatory Potential of Diet, Weight Gain, and Incidence of Overweight/Obesity: The SUN Cohort," *Obesity* 25, no. 6 (June 2017): 997–1005, https://doi.org/10.1002/oby.21833.

11. R. Monteiro and I. Azevedo, "Chronic Inflammation in Obesity and the Metabolic Syndrome," *Mediators of Inflammation* 2010, article ID 289645 (2010), https://doi.org/10.1155/2010/289645.

Chapter 8: *Staying Healthy in a Toxic World: A Guide to Beating Environmental Toxins*

1. "Electric & Magnetic Fields," NIH National Institute of Environmental Health Sciences, accessed August 16, 2018, https://www.niehs.nih.gov/health/topics/agents/emf.

2. N. Borhani, F. Rajaei, Z. Salehi, et al., "Analysis of DNA Fragmentation in Mouse Embryos Exposed to an Extremely Low-Frequency Electromagnetic Field," *Electromagnetic Biology and Medicine* 30, no. 4 (December 2011): 246–52, https://doi.org/10.3109/15368378.2011.589556.

3. A. Asghari, A. A. Khaki, A. Rajabzadeh, et al., "A Review on Electromagnetic Fields (EMFs) and the Reproductive System," *Electronic Physician* 8, no. 7 (July 2016): 2655–62, https://doi.org/10.19082/2655.

4. J. K. Grayson, "Radiation Exposure, Socioeconomic Status, and Brain Tumor Risk in the US Air Force: A Nested Case-Control Study," *American Journal of Epidemiology* 143, no. 5 (March 1, 1996): 480–86.

5. M. Havas, "Dirty Electricity Elevates Blood Sugar Among Electrically Sensitive Diabetics and May Explain Brittle Diabetes," *Electromagnetic Biology and Medicine* 27, no. 2 (2008): 135–46, https://doi/org/10.1080/15368370802072075.

6. S. Milham, "Evidence That Dirty Electricity Is Causing the Worldwide Epidemics of Obesity and Diabetes," *Electromagnetic Biology and Medicine* 33, no. 1 (June 2013), https://doi.org/10.3109/15368378.2013.783853.

7. M. L. Pall, "Microwave Frequency Electromagnetic Fields (EMFs) Produce Widespread Neuropsychiatric Effects Including Depression," *Journal of Chemical Neuroanatomy* 75, pt. B (September 2016): 43–51, https://doi.org/10.1016/j.jchemneu.2015.08.001.

8. I. Yakymenko, E. Sidorik, S. Kyrylenko, et al., "Long-Term Exposure to Microwave Radiation Provokes Cancer Growth: Evidences from Radars and Mobile Communication Systems," *Experimental Oncology* 33, no. 2 (June 2011): 62–70.

9. World Health Organization (WHO), *Establishing a Dialogue on Risks from Electromagnetic Fields.* (Geneva: Radiation and Environmental Health Department of Protection of the

Human Environment WHO, 2002), accessed August 27, 2018, http://apps.who.int/iris/bitstream/handle/10665/42543/9241545712_eng.pdf?sequence=1&isAllowed=y.

10. L. Hardell and M. Carlberg, "Mobile Phone and Cordless Phone Use and the Risk for Glioma—Analysis of Pooled Case-Control Studies in Sweden, 1997–2003 and 2007–2009," *Pathophysiology* 22, no. 1 (March 2015): 1–13, https://doi.org/10.1016/j.pathophys.2014.10.001.

11. L. Hardell, A. Näsman, A. Påhlson, et al., "Use of Cellular Telephones and the Risk for Brain Tumours: A Case-Control Study," *International Journal of Oncology* 15, no. 1 (July1999): 113–16.

12. L. Hardell, K. H. Mild, and M. Carlberg, "Further Aspects on Cellular and Cordless Telephones and Brain Tumours," *International Journal of Oncology* 22, no 2 (2003): 399–407, accessed August 16, 2018, http://avaate.org/IMG/pdf/Int_J_Oncol_2003_22_399.pdf.

13. I. N. Fossum, L. T. Nordnes, S. S. Storemark, et al., "The Association Between Use of Electronic Media in Bed Before Going to Sleep and Insomnia Symptoms, Daytime Sleepiness, Morningness, and Chronotype," *Behavioral Sleep Medicine* 12, no. 5 (2014): 343–57, https://doi.org/10.1080/15402002.2013.819468.

14. L. Giuliani and M. Soffritti, eds., *Non-thermal Effects and Mechanisms of Interaction Between Electromagnetic Fields and Living Matter,* vol. 5, *European Journal of Oncology* (Bologna, Italy: National Institute for the Study and Control of Cancer and Environmental Diseases, 2010).

15. S. La Vignera, R. A. Condorelli, E. Vicari, et al., "Effects of the Exposure to Mobile Phones on Male Reproduction: A Review of the Literature," *Journal of Andrology* 33, no. 3 (May 2012): 350–56, https://doi.org/10.2164/jandrol.111.014373.

16. S. Bhagat, S. Varshney, S. Bist, et al., "Effects of Chronic Exposure to Mobile Phones Electromagnetic Fields on Inner Ear," *Internet Journal of Otorhinolaryngology* 14, no. 2 (2012), accessed October 25, 2018, https://print.ispub.com/api/0/ispub-article/14261.

17. "iPhone 6 SAR: Radiation Levels & Separation Distance," Electromagnetic Radiation Safety, September 29, 2015, http://www.saferemr.com/search?q=sar.

18. Simon Sinek, "Addiction to Technology Is Ruining Lives," YouTube video, 4:02, from an interview on *Inside Quest,* accessed August 16, 2018, https://www.youtube.com/watch?v=sL8AsaEJDdo.

19. "Blue Light Has a Dark Side," Harvard Health Publishing (Harvard Medical School), last updated August 13, 2018, https://www.health.harvard.edu/staying-healthy/blue-light-has-a-dark-side.

20. C. A. A. Zamfir, C. R. Popescu, and D. C. Gheorghe, "Melatonin and Cancer," *Journal of Medicine and Life* 7, no. 3 (September 2014): 373–74.

21. S. M. J. Mortazavi, S. A. Mortazavi, P. Habibzadeh, et al., "Is It Blue Light or Increased Electromagnetic Fields Which Affects the Circadian Rhythm in People Who Use Smartphones at Night," *Iranian Journal of Public Health* 45, no. 3 (March 2016): 405–06.

22. M. Figueiro, B. Wood, B. Plitnick, et al., "The Impact of Light from Computer Monitors on Melatonin Levels in College Students," *Neuro Endocrinology Letters* 32, no. 2 (2011): 158–63.

23. K. Burkhart and J. R. Phelps, "Amber Lenses to Block Blue Light and Improve Sleep: A Randomized Trial," *Chronobiology International* 26, no. 6 (2009): 1602–12.

24. M. H. Ward, T. M. deKok, P. Levallois, et al., "Workgroup Report: Drinking-Water Nitrate and Health—Recent Findings and Research Needs," *Environmental Health Perspectives* 113, no. 11 (November 2005): 1607–14.

25. L. T. Stayner, K. Almberg, R. Jones, et al., "Atrazine and Nitrate in Drinking Water and the Risk of Preterm Delivery and Low Birth Weight in Four Midwestern States," *Environmental Research* 152 (January 2017): 294–303, https://doi.org/10.1016/j.envres.2016.10.022.

26. J. D. Brender, K. Almberg, R. Jones, et al., "Prenatal Nitrate Intake from Drinking Water and Selected Birth Defects in Offspring of Participants in the National Birth Defects Prevention Study," *Environmental Health Perspectives* 121, no. 9 (January 2013): 1083–89, https://doi.org/10.1289/ehp.1206249.

27. R. R. Jones, P. J. Weyer, C. T. DellaValle, et al., "Nitrate from Drinking Water and Diet and Bladder Cancer Among Postmenopausal Women in Iowa," *Environmental Health Perspectives* 124, no. 11 (June 2016): 1751–58, https://doi.org/10.1289/EHP191.

28. US Geological Survey, *USGS Technical Announcement: Widely Used Herbicide Commonly Found in Rain and Streams in the Mississippi River Basin* (Reston, VA: US Department of the Interior/USGS, 2011).

29. US Environmental Protection Agency, *Technical Factsheet on: Glyphosate*, available at http://www.epa.gov/safewater/pdfs/factsheets/soc/tech/glyphosa.pdf.

30. T. Bøhn, M. Cuhra, T. Traavik, et al., "Compositional Differences in Soybeans on the Market: Glyphosate Accumulates in Roundup Ready GM Soybeans," *Food Chemistry* 153 (June 2014): 207–15, https://doi.org/10.1016/j.foodchem.2013.12.054.

31. J. F. Acquavella, B. H. Alexander, J. S. Mandel, et al., "Glyphosate Biomonitoring for Farmers and Their Families: Results from the Farm Family Exposure Study," *Environmental Health Perspectives* 112, no. 3 (2004): 321–26, http://www.ncbi.nlm.nih.gov/pmc/articles/PMC1241861.

32. K. Z. Guyton, D. Loomis, Y. Grosse, et al., "Carcinogenicity of Tetrachlorvinphos, Parathion, Malathion, Diazinon & Glyphosate," *Lancet Oncology* 16, no. 5 (May 2015): 490–91, https://doi.org/10.1016/S1470-2045(15)70134-8.

33. D. Brandli and S. Reinacher, "Herbicides Found in Human Urine," *Ithaka Journal* 1 (2012): 270–72, http://www.ithaka-journal.net/druckversionen/e052012-herbicides-urine.pdf.

34. J. P. S. Cabral, "Water Microbiology, Bacterial Pathogens and Water," *International Journal of Environmental Research and Public Health* 7, no. 10 (2010): 3657–703, https://doi.org/10.3390/ijerph7103657.

35. R. Bain, R. Cronk, J. Wright, et al., "Fecal Contamination of Drinking-Water in Low- and Middle-Income Countries: A Systematic Review and Meta-analysis," *PLoS Medicine* 11, no. 5 (2014): e1001644, https://doi.org/10.1371/journal.pmed.1001644.

36. M. N. Babič, N. Grunde-Cimerman, M. Vargha, et al., "Fungal Contaminants in Drinking Water Regulation? A Tale of Ecology, Exposure, Purification and Clinical Relevance," *International Journal of Environmental Research and Public Health* 14, no. 6 (2017): 636, https://doi.org/10.3390/ijerph14060636.

37. H. M. Murphy, K. M. Thomas, D. T. Medeiros, et al., "Estimating the Number of Cases of Acute Gastrointestinal Illness (AGI) Associated with Canadian Municipal Drinking Water Systems," *Epidemiology and Infection* 144, no. 7 (May 2016): 1371–85, https://doi.org/10.1017/S0950268815002083.

38. "Glossary," EWG's Healthy Living: Home Guide, accessed August 16, 2018, https://www.ewg.org/healthyhomeguide/glossary/#.W3X4xpNKii4.

39. A. L. Simmons, J. J. Schleinger, and B. E. Corkey, "What Are We Putting in Our Food That Is Making Us Fat? Food Additives, Contaminants, and Other Putative Con-

tributors to Obesity," *Current Obesity Reports* 3, no. 2 (June 2014): 273–85, https://doi
.org/10.1007/s13679-014-0094-y.

40.   T. Schettler, J. Stein, F. Reich, et al., *In Harm's Way: Toxic Threats to Child Development*
(Cambridge, MA: Greater Boston Physicians for Social Responsibility, 2000), accessed
August 16, 2018, http://action.psr.org/site/DocServer/ihwcomplete.pdf?docID=5131.

41.   J. S. A. de Araujo, I. F. Delgaso, and F. J. R. Paumgartten, "Glyphosate and Adverse
Pregnancy Outcomes, a Systematic Review Of Observational Studies," *BMC Public
Health* 16 (2016): 472, https://doi.org/10.1186/s12889-016-3153-3.

42.   "Monsanto Ordered to Pay $289 Million in Roundup Cancer Trial," *New York Times,*
August 10, 2018, https://www.nytimes.com/2018/08/10/business/monsanto-roundup
-cancer-trial.html.

43.   J. Bloom, "MIT Researcher: Glyphosate Will Cause Half of All Children to Be Au-
tistic by 2025. Yeah, Sure," American Council of Science and Health, June 7, 2017,
https://www.acsh.org/news/2017/06/07/mit-researcher-glyphosate-will-cause-half
-all-children-be-autistic-2025-yeah-sure-11337.

44.   National Institute for Occupational Safety and Health, "Health Hazard Evaluation Report (HETA 83-085-1757)," accessed August 16, 2018, https://www.cdc.gov/niosh/
hhe/reports/pdfs/83-85-1757.pdf?id=10.26616/NIOSHEETA830851757.

45.   M. B. Abou-Donia, A. M. Dechkovskaia, L. B. Goldstein, et al., "Co-exposure to Pyr-
idostigmine Bromide, DEET, and/or Permethrin Causes Sensorimotor Deficit and Al-
terations in Brain Acetylcholinesterase Activity," *Pharmacology, Biochemistry and Behavior*
77, no. 2 (February 2004): 253–62.

46.   A. Abdel-Rahman, A. M. Dechkovskaia, L. B. Goldstein, et al., "Neurological Defi-
cits Induced by Malathion, DEET, and Permethrin, Alone or in Combination in Adult
Rats," *Journal of Toxicology and Environmental Health Part A* 67, no. 4 (February 2004):
331–56.

Chapter 9: The Keys to an Abundant Life

1.   Sonja Lyubomirsky, *The How of Happiness: A New Approach to Getting the Life You Want*
(New York: Penguin Press, 2008).

2.   J. Helliwell, R. Layard, and J. Sachs, eds., *World Happiness Report,* published April 2, 2012,
accessed August 18, 2018, http://documents.latimes.com/world-happiness-report.

3.   J. Helliwell, R. Layard, and J. Sachs, eds., *World Happiness Report 2017* (New York: Sustainable Development Solutions Network, 2017), accessed August 18, 2018, https://
s3.amazonaws.com/happiness-report/2017/HR17.pdf.

4.   "Forgiveness: Your Health Depends on It," Johns Hopkins Medicine, accessed August 18, 2018, www.hopkinsmedicine.org/health/healthy_aging/healthy_connections/
forgiveness-your-health-depends-on-it.

5.   Ibid.

6.   L. T. Toussaint, A. D. Owen, A. Cheadle, "Forgive to Live: Forgiveness, Health, and
Longevity," *Journal of Behavioral Medicine* 35, no. 4 (August 2012): 375–86.

7.   C. Romero, L. C. Friedman, M. Kalidas, et al., "Self-Forgiveness, Spirituality, and Psychological Adjustment in Women with Breast Cancer," *Journal of Behavioral Medicine* 29,
no. 1 (February 2006): 29–36.

8.   L. Legault, T. Al-Khindi, and M. Inzlicht, "Preserving Integrity in the Face of Performance Threat: Self-Affirmation Enhances Neurophysiological Responsiveness

to Errors," *Psychological Science* 23, no. 12 (2012): 1455–60, https://doi.org/10.1177/0956797612448483.

9. L. Collier, "Why We Cry: New Research Is Opening Eyes to the Psychology of Tears," *Monitor on Psychology* 45, no. 2 (February 2014): 47.

10. A. Gračanin, L. M. Bylsma, and A. J. J. M. Vingerhoets, "Is Crying a Self-Soothing Behavior?" *Frontiers in Psychology* 5 (May 2014): 502, https://doi.org/10.3389/fpsyg.2014.00502.

11. American Institute of Stress, accessed August 18, 2018, www.stress.org/emotional-and-social-support.

12. C. Edson Jr., P. Ferrucci, and M. Dufy, "Facebook Use, Envy, and Depression Among College Students: Is Facebooking Depressing?" *Computers in Human Behavior* 43 (February 2015): 139–46, https://doi.org/10.1016/j.chb.2014.10.053.

13. H. G. Koenig, "Religion, Spirituality, and Health: The Research and Clinical Implications," *ISRN Psychiatry* 2012, article 278730 (2012), http://doi.org/10.5402/2012/278730.

14. A. Al-Thaqui, F. Al-Sultan, A. Al-Zahrani, et al., "Brain Training Games Enhance Cognitive Function in Healthy Subjects," *Medical Science Monitor Basic Research* 24 (April 20, 2018): 63–69.

15. R. Nouchi, Y. Taki, H. Takeuchi, et al., "Brain Training Game Boosts Executive Functions, Working Memory and Processing Speed in the Young Adults: A Randomized Controlled Trial," *PLoS ONE* 8, no. 2 (2013): e55518, https://doi.org/10.1371/journal.pone.0055518.

16. J. Vlahos, "Is Sitting a Lethal Activity?" *New York Times Magazine,* April 14, 2011, https://www.nytimes.com/2011/04/17/magazine/mag-17sitting-t.html.

17. L. F. M. Rezende, T. H. Sá, G. I. Mielke, et al., "All-Cause Mortality Attributable to Sitting Time: Analysis of 54 Countries Worldwide," *American Journal of Preventive Medicine* 51, no. 2 (August 2016): 253–63, https://doi.org/10.1016/j.amepre.2016.01.022.

18. Dan Buettner, "How to Live to Be 100+," filmed September 2009, TED video, 19:25, accessed August 18, 2018, https://www.ted.com/talks/dan_buettner_how_to_live_to_be_100.

19. A. MacMillan, "How Exercise May Help Protect Your Brain from Cognitive Decline and Dementia," *Time,* February 16, 2018, http://time.com/5162477/exercise-risk-dementia.

The Essential Exercise Program

1. "A Few 30 Second Sprints as Beneficial as Hour-Long Jog," *ScienceDaily,* June 2, 2005, www.sciencedaily.com/releases/2005/06/050602113341.htm.

2. K. A. Stokes, D. Sykes, K. L. Gilbert, et al., "Brief, High Intensity Exercise Alters Serum Ghrelin and Growth Hormone Concentrations but Not IGF-I, IGF-II or IGF-I Bioactivity," *Growth Hormone IGF Research* 20, no. 4 (August 2010): 289–94, https://doi.org/10.1016/j.ghir.2010.03.004.

3. C. Werner, M. Hauser, K. Schirra, et al., "High Intensity Interval Training Activates Telomerase and Reduces P53 Expression," accessed August 24, 2018, http://spo.escardio.org/eslides/view.aspx?eevtid=54&fp=5229.

4. K. Van Proeyen, K. Szlufcik, H. Nielens, et al., "Training in the Fasted State Improves Glucose Tolerance During Fat-Rich Diet," *Journal of Physiology* 588, no. 21 (November 1, 2010): 4289–302, https://doi.org/10.1113/jphysiol.2010.196493.

RECOMMENDED RESOURCES

These resources will help you on your journey as you follow the guidelines outlined in the Essential Oils Diet. If you have any questions or a testimonial you'd like to share, please contact us at Support@ NaturalLivingFamily.com. We always love to read the healing stories that flow through our inbox, telling us how bioactive-rich foods and essential oils have changed people's lives!

ESSENTIAL OILS DIET SUCCESS PACKAGE (FREE GIFT)
- Shopping tour, exercise and recipe demo videos
- Starter checklists, shopping guides, meal plans, and more
- Essential Fast Track and Essential Lifestyle approved
- **EssentialOilsDiet.com**

Essential Oils Resources

ESSENTIAL OILS FOR ABUNDANT LIVING MASTER CLASS
- Free viewing of our ten-part video series to help you use essential oils the right way
- **EssentialOilsForAbundantLiving.com**

THE HEALING POWER OF ESSENTIAL OILS BOOK
- With more than 150 effective recipes and natural remedies
- **HealingPowerOfEssentialOils.com**

DR. Z'S ESSENTIAL OILS CLUB
- Essential oils education membership
- **EssentialOilsClub.info**

Detox Resources

TOXIC-FREE HEALTHY HOME MAKEOVER TOUR
- Free viewing of our five-part video series showing you how we've detoxed our home
- **NaturalLivingFamily.com/HomeMakeover**

NATURAL LIVING PROGRAMS
- Online courses to help you cook healthy food, garden organically, exercise the right way, and live a healthy life
- **NaturalLivingFamily.com/Programs**

ESSENTIAL PRODUCTS
- **NaturalLivingFamily.com/how-to-be-healthy/**—for a list of all the products, supplements, books, and educational resources we recommend.
- Air Doctor—the best, most affordable (portable) air-purification system we have ever used. Learn how you can get a special Natural Living Family group-buy discount at **NaturalLivingFamily.com/AirDr.**
- **Amazon.com**—an excellent resource for containers to hold your oil blends, including lotion dispensers, spritz bottles, and even stick deodorant containers.
- Annmarie Skin Care—when you can't make DIY skincare products, we recommend Annmarie Skin Care. We have used this completely natural, nontoxic skin care line for years. Learn more at **NaturalLivingFamily.com/Annmarie.**
- Living Fuel SuperGreens—the supermeal that you can drink. When we want to boost our nutrition and shed

stubborn weight, Living Fuel is our go-to. Check it out at **NaturalLivingFamily.com/LivingFuel.**

- MyGreenFills—we only know of one chemical-free, nontoxic laundry solution: MyGreenFills. Trust us, as a family of six, we do fifteen loads a week! Learn more at **NaturalLivingFamily.com/MyGreenFills.**
- Thrive Market—a membership community that uses the power of direct buying to ship the world's best healthy food and natural products at wholesale prices. To join and get a special discount, visit **NaturalLivingFamily.com/Thrive.**
- Trim Healthy Mama—our friends Pearl and Serene have created some of the healthiest foods and body-care products on the Internet. Check out what they offer by visiting **NaturalLivingFamily.com/TrimHealthyMama.**
- Wholetones—sold out on QVC in eight minutes! Our friend and Grammy-award-winning musician Michael Tyrrell created Wholetones—instrumental music that uses special frequencies to help restore the mind, body, and soul. Learn more at **NaturalLivingFamily.com/Wholetones.**

Aromatherapy Reference Books, Texts, and Certification Courses

- Atlantic Institute of Aromatherapy: AtlanticInstitute.com
- Buckle, Jane. *Clinical Aromatherapy: Essential Oils in Healthcare,* 3rd ed. (St. Louis, MO: Churchill Livingstone, 2014).
- Price, Len, and Shirley Price. *Understanding Hydrolats: The Specific Hydrosols for Aromatherapy: A Guide for Health Professionals*. (London: Churchill Livingstone, 2004).
- Price, Shirley, and Len Price. *Aromatherapy for Health Professionals,* 4th ed. (London: Churchill Livingstone, 2011).
- Rose, Jeanne. *375 Essential Oils and Hydrosols* (Berkeley, CA: Frog, 1999).
- Sheppard-Hanger, Sylla. *The Aromatherapy Practitioner Reference Manual,* 2 vols. (Tampa, FL: Atlantic Institute of Aromatherapy, 1997).

- Tisserand, Robert, and Rodney Young. *Essential Oil Safety: A Guide for Health Care Professionals,* 2nd ed. (London: Churchill Livingstone, 2013).

Environmental Working Group Health and Safety Guides

- EWG's Skin Deep Cosmetics Database: EWG.org/skindeep
- EWG's Guide to Healthy Cleaning: EWG.org/guides/cleaners
- EWG's Food Scores: EWG.org/foodscores

INDEX

Wraps, Brown Rice Veggie, with Pesto, 238

ABOUT THE AUTHORS

The author of the national bestseller *The Healing Power of Essential Oils*, Dr. Eric Zielinski has pioneered natural living and biblical health education since 2003. Trained as an aromatherapist, public health researcher, and chiropractor, Dr. Z started DrEricZ.com (now Natural LivingFamily.com) in 2014 with his wife, Sabrina Ann, to help people learn how to safely and effectively use natural remedies such as essential oils.

Sabrina Ann Zielinski is a certified group fitness instructor, health coach, lactation consultant, and a natural health guru. The mastermind behind the allergy-friendly food recipes and do-it-yourself remedies featured on their website and in this book, she's known as "Mama Z" to many mamas who are looking for natural ways to care for their families.

Now visited by more than seven million natural health seekers every year, NaturalLivingFamily.com has rapidly become the number one online source for biblical health and non-branded essential oils education.

The Zs live in Atlanta with their four children.

Some Enchanted Evening

CHRISTINA DODD

WILLIAM MORROW
An Imprint of HarperCollins*Publishers*

This is a work of fiction. The characters, incidents, and
dialogue are products of the author's imagination
and are not to be construed as real. Any resemblance to
actual events or persons, living or dead, is entirely coincidental.

HarperCollins books may be purchased for educational, business, or
sales promotional use. For information please write: Special Markets
Department, HarperCollins Publishers Inc., 10 East 53rd Street,
New York, NY 10022.

FIRST EDITION

Designed by Paula Russell Szafranski

Printed on acid-free paper

Library of Congress Cataloging-in-Publication Data

Dodd, Christina.
  Some enchanted evening / by Christina Dodd.—1st ed.
    p. cm.
  ISBN 0-06-056124-6 (alk. paper)
  1. Kings and rulers—Succession—Fiction. 2. Princesses—Fiction. 3. Nobil-
ity—Fiction. 4. Scotland—Fiction. I. Title.

PS3554.O3175S66 2004
813'.54—dc22   2003064937

04 05 06 07 08 WBC/RRD 10 9 8 7 6 5 4 3 2 1